ASHP's **Safety** and **Quality PEARLS**

Melodi J. McNeil, R.Ph., MS
Director, Regulatory Intelligence
Global Pharmaceutical Regulatory
  and Medical Sciences
Abbott Laboratories
Rockville, Maryland

American Society of Health-System Pharmacists®
Bethesda, Maryland

Any correspondence regarding this publication should be sent to the publisher, American Society of Health-System Pharmacists, 7272 Wisconsin Avenue, Bethesda, MD 20814, attention: Special Publishing.

The information presented herein reflects the opinions of the contributors and advisors. It should not be interpreted as an official policy of ASHP or as an endorsement of any product.

Because of ongoing research and improvements in technology, the information and its applications contained in this text are constantly evolving and are subject to the professional judgment and interpretation of the practitioner due to the uniqueness of a clinical situation. The editors, contributors, and ASHP have made reasonable efforts to ensure the accuracy and appropriateness of the information presented in this document. However, any user of this information is advised that the editors, contributors, advisors, and ASHP are not responsible for the continued currency of the information, for any errors or omissions, and/or for any consequences arising from the use of the information in the document in any and all practice settings. Any reader of this document is cautioned that ASHP makes no representation, guarantee, or warranty, express or implied, as to the accuracy and appropriateness of the information contained in this document and specifically disclaims any liability to any party for the accuracy and/or completeness of the material or for any damages arising out of the use or non-use of any of the information contained in this document.

Director, Special Publishing: Jack Bruggeman
Senior Editorial Project Manager: Dana Battaglia
Project Editor: Kristin Eckles
Cover Design: DeVall Advertising
Page Design: David Wade and Carol Barrer

Library of Congress Cataloging-in-Publication Data

ASHP's safety and quality pearls / [edited by] Melodi J. McNeil.
     p. ; cm.
  A selection of presentations from a "Safety and Quality Pearls" session held at the 2006 ASHP Midyear Clinical Meeting in Anaheim, Calif.
  Includes bibliographical references and index.
  ISBN 978-1-58528-197-8
1. Hospital pharmacies--Quality control--Congresses. 2. Drugs--Standards--Congresses. I. McNeil, Melodi J. II. American Society of Health-System Pharmacists. III. ASHP Midyear Clinical Meeting (41st : 2006 : Anaheim, Calif.) IV. Title: Safety and quality pearls. V. Title: American Society of Health-System Pharmacists' safety and quality pearls.
  [DNLM: 1. Pharmacy Service, Hospital--standards--Congresses. 2. Drug Therapy--standards--Congresses. 3. Medication Errors--prevention & control--Congresses. 4. Pharmacy Service, Hospital--organization & administration--Congresses. 5. Safety Management--organization & administration--Congresses. WX 179 A827 2008]

  RA975.5.P5A84 2008
  362.17'82--dc22

                             2008005931

ISBN: 978-1-58528-197-8

Table of Contents

Part 3: Tools

Acknowledgment

ASHP wishes to thank Abbott Laboratories for its support of this project, in the form of Ms. McNeil's time.

Preface

Is there any pharmacist who has *not* experienced the sinking sensation that comes from being involved in a medication error* (regardless of whether a patient was harmed as a result)?

In 1999 the Institute of Medicine (IOM) significantly elevated the public profile of medication errors with the publication of a report entitled, "To Err is Human: Building a Safer Health System." Based on estimates from two other, previously conducted studies, the IOM extrapolated that between 44,000 and 98,000 people die annually in hospitals as a result of medical errors[1] and described a comprehensive strategy by which stakeholders (healthcare professionals, the pharmaceutical industry, patients, and others) can reduce preventable medical errors.

Subsequently (in 2001), the IOM published a report on the quality† of care delivered in the U.S. Health System entitled, "Crossing the Quality Chasm: A New Health System for the 21st Century." Among this report's findings were that "...between the healthcare that we now have and the healthcare that we could have lies not just a gap, but a chasm."[2] The report's authors attributed this chasm to the growing complexity of healthcare, an inability of the healthcare delivery system to translate knowledge into practice, and a healthcare system overly focused on acute, episodic care needs.[2]

Most recently, IOM studied the prevalence of medication errors and summarized its findings in a 2006 report entitled, "Preventing Medication Errors." Here, the IOM found that medication errors are both common (especially at the prescribing and administration stages of the medication process) and costly.[3] The IOM conservatively estimated that there are at least 400,000 medication errors in U.S. hospitals each year, at a cost of about $8,750 per event or $3.5 billion annually.[3]

Regardless of whether one agrees with these reports' specific conclusions or how the statistics in these reports were calculated, there is general agreement with the reports' overall conclusion that medication errors and suboptimal medical care are a significant public health concern. Debates about the validity of the numbers obscure the more significant point, which is that patients are experiencing substantial morbidity and mortality due to a flawed health system.[6]

Pharmacists' duties have undergone a tremendous evolution from the days when we simply dispensed medications accurately in response to a prescriber's valid prescription. Today, pharmacists, still ultimately responsible for dispensing medications accurately, are also expected to be purveyors of *rational* drug therapy. This evolution, closely associated with patient benefit—numerous studies have shown that increased pharmacist involvement in patient care is associated with improved health outcomes—also means increased opportunities for pharmacists to positively influence the multiple steps in the medication dispensing and administration process. Not surprisingly then, the pharmacy profession (pharmacists in particular) is a key stakeholder in many of the recommendations made in the IOM reports cited above.

The 2006 ASHP Midyear Clinical Meeting included the premiere of a session entitled, "Safety and Quality Pearls." This session was conceived as a response to the rather grim portrait of the U.S. healthcare system painted by the three IOM reports. In particular, I wanted to see if it was possible to convene a forum that would confirm my suspicions, namely that America's health-system pharmacists were not all passively accepting and/or part of the dismal reality painted by the IOM reports, but were instead making real, robust, and successful attempts to address the system breakdowns that might be implicated in errors or less than quality care in their institutions. I also wanted to move beyond *general* statements of problems and *general* recommendations to *specific*, practical advice on solutions from the ground zero perspective of pharmacists and technicians who are living with the realities of these medication use issues every day.

---

*Medication errors, a subset of medical errors, are preventable events that may cause or lead to inappropriate medication use or patient harm while the medication is in the control of the healthcare professional, patient, or consumer.[4]

†Quality is defined as the degree to which health services for individuals and populations increase the likelihood of desired health outcomes and are consistent with current professional knowledge.[2]

The Safety and Quality Pearls session was patterned after the popular Clinical, Informatics, and Management Pearls programs routinely held at the Midyear Clinical Meeting. The goal of each presentation in a Pearls session is to convey a single idea, concept, or fact (that may not be widely known, understood, published, or taught) in a very short amount of time. Specifically, each presenter in the Safety and Quality Pearls program had five minutes (strictly enforced with the help of a large traffic light) to describe a single thing that had been done in his or her health-system pharmacy to enhance patient safety[‡] or the quality of patient care.

This book pulls together in one place 20 of the original 27 presentations. Pearls are presented in three categories: compliance with national quality standards and/or clinical guidelines, technology/devices, and quality improvement tools. Many of the Pearls have been expanded (for example, with updated data) for publication, so even if you attended this session at the 2006 Midyear, this book will offer a fresh perspective on the Pearls. If you've ever attended a Pearls session, you know they are intentionally more informal and lighthearted than the other, traditional Midyear presentations. Because there is a different speaker at the podium approximately every five minutes or so, the Pearls sessions are a "Short Attention Span Theater" of sorts. We've tried to retain that fun spirit for the book.

I'm also pleased with the diversity of the Pearls presented in this collection. The authors represent both large and small health systems; public and private institutions; academic medical centers; government healthcare facilities; and small, outpatient clinics. All of the Pearls are pharmacy-centric, but you'll notice that many required multidisciplinary effort to implement. In short, we've tried to include something of relevance for as many audiences as possible. Our hope is that reading these Pearls will inspire you to attempt similar interventions in your own institutions, if you haven't already done so. We've made it a point to provide contact information for each contributor, to facilitate your ability to get more information if you do decide to try any of the ideas described here.

As some of the more alarming statistics from the IOM reports make their way into scientific journals and the lay media, it is easy to get discouraged about the state of the U.S. healthcare system. While this collection of Pearls is certainly no panacea, it does represent a source of encouragement, in that it showcases a collection of health-system pharmacies whose staff is actively involved in working to improve patient care. Of course, it's also exciting to contemplate the idea that this book likely represents only a fraction of the programs aimed at increasing both the safety and the quality of medication use that are being conceived and executed in health-system pharmacies around the country.

The topic of safe and appropriate medication use has the potential to personally affect us all, whether we are healthcare professionals, patients, or the family members of patients. Though I was a practicing pharmacist for several years, today I work in the pharmaceutical industry. I remain particularly interested in the pharmacy profession's efforts to improve patient care, and I believe by working together we can achieve the "Safer Health System" promised by the title of the 1999 IOM report. In the meantime, my hope is that this book will become a resource for those healthcare professionals who are contemplating safety and quality improvements in their health systems.

Melodi J. McNeil, R.Ph., MS
Director, Regulatory Intelligence
Global Pharmaceutical Regulatory and Medical Sciences
Abbott Laboratories
melodi.mcneil@abbott.com

[‡]Safety is defined as the freedom from accidental injury.[5]

References

1. Institute of Medicine. *To Err is Human: Building a Safer Health System*: November 1999. Report Brief. Available at: http://www.iom.edu/Object.File/Master/4/117/ToErr-8pager.pdf. Accessed September 11, 2007.

2. Institute of Medicine. *Crossing the Quality Chasm: A New Health System for the 21st Century:* March 2001. Report Brief. Available at: http://www.iom.edu/Object.File/Master/27/184/Chasm-8pager.pdf. Accessed September 11, 2007.

3. Institute of Medicine. *Preventing Medication Errors:* July 2006. Report Brief. Available at: http://www.iom.edu/Object.File/Master/35/943/medication%20errors%20new.pdf. Accessed September 11, 2007.

4. National Coordinating Council for Medication Error Reporting and Prevention. Available at: http://www.nccmerp.org/aboutMedErrors.html. Accessed September 11, 2007.

5. Institute of Medicine. *To Err is Human: Building a Safer Health System:* 2000. Washington, DC: National Academy of Sciences; 2000.

6. Dotseth M. Testimony presented at: National Summit on Medical Errors and Patient Safety Research; September 11, 2000; Washington, DC. Available at: www.quic.gov/summit/wdotseth1.htm. Accessed September 11, 2007.

Contributors

Antonia Alafris, BS, Pharm.D., CGP
Associate Director
Pharmacotherapy Services and Pharmacy Residency Programs
Department of Pharmacy
Kingsbrook Jewish Medical Center
Brooklyn, New York
Aalafris@aol.com

Sarah Barber, Pharm.D.
Children's Hospitals and Clinics of Minnesota
Clinical Staff Pharmacist and Pharmacist-In-Charge
Shriners Hospital for Children
St. Paul, Minnesota
sarah.barber@childrensmn.org

Sharon R. Baty, Pharm.D.
Cardiology Clinical Specialist
Department of Pharmacy
Huntsville Hospital
Huntsville, Alabama
sharo045@hhsys.org

Jered B. Bauer, Pharm.D.
Director, Clinical Services
Operations Department
Broadlane
Dallas, Texas
jered.bauer@broadlane.com

Sandra L. Chase, BS, Pharm.D., FMPA
Cardiopulmonary Clinical Specialist
Spectrum Health
Grand Rapids, Michigan
Adjunct Assistant Professor of Pharmacy
Ferris State University College of Pharmacy
Big Rapids, Michigan
SChase731@aol.com

Henry Cohen, BS, MS, Pharm.D., FCCM, BCPP, CGP
Associate Professor of Pharmacy Practice
Arnold & Marie Schwartz College of Pharmacy and Health Sciences
Long Island University
Chief Pharmacotherapy Officer
Director of Pharmacy Residency Programs (PGY-1 and PGY-2)
Kingsbrook Jewish Medical Center
Department of Pharmacy Services
Brooklyn, New York
HCohenliu@aol.com

Ernest J. Dole, Pharm.D., R.Ph.
Pharmaceutical Care Coordinator
ABQHealth Partners
Albuquerque, New Mexico
ERNEST.DOLE@abqhp.com

Michele Durda, Pharm.D.
Medication Safety/Drug Utilization Pharmacist
Huntsville Hospital
Huntsville, Alabama
miche118@hhsys.org

Kelly C. A. Ervin, CPhT.
Pharmacy Quality Data Analyst
Drug Use and Disease State Management Program
Department of Pharmacy and Therapeutics
University of Pittsburgh Medical Center
Pittsburgh, Pennsylvania
ErvinKC@upmc.edu

Rebecca Garner, Pharm.D., BCPS, LCDR
U.S. Public Health Service
Phoenix Indian Medical Center
Phoenix, Arizona
Rebecca.Garner@ihs.gov

Karen Suchanek Hudmon, Dr.P.H., MS, R.Ph.
Associate Professor, Department of Pharmacy Practice
Purdue University School of Pharmacy & Pharmaceutical Sciences
Research Affiliate, Department of Chronic Disease Epidemiology
Yale University School of Public Health
Assistant Clinical Professor, Department of Clinical Pharmacy
University of California San Francisco School of Pharmacy
khudmon@purdue.edu

Heather Myers Huentelman, Pharm.D., BCPS
LT, U.S. Public Health Service
Phoenix Indian Medical Center
Phoenix, Arizona
heather.huentelman@ihs.gov

Kathleen Johnston, RN, MSN
Quality Improvement Specialist
Quality Department
Spectrum Health
Grand Rapids, Michigan
Big Rapids, Michigan
Kathleen.Johnston@Spectrumhealth.org

Joanne G. Kowiatek, R.Ph., MPM
Adjunct Assistant Professor of Pharmacy and Therapeutics
University of Pittsburgh School of Pharmacy
Pharmacy Manager, Medication Patient Safety
University of Pittsburgh Medical Center
Pittsburgh, Pennsylvania
KowiatekJG@upmc.edu

Connie Larson, Pharm.D.
Medication Safety Officer
Assistant Director, Safety and Quality
Hospital Pharmacy Services
University of Illinois Medical Center at Chicago
Clinical Assistant Professor
Department of Pharmacy Practice
University of Illinois at Chicago College of Pharmacy
Chicago, Illinois
CLarson@uic.edu

Todd Lemke, Pharm.D., CDE
Director of Pharmacy Services
Paynesville Area Health Care System
Paynesville, Minnesota
tlemke@pahcs.com

David Merryfield, R.Ph.
Director, Clinical Pharmacy Programs
Sentara Healthcare
Norfolk, Virginia
dwmerryf@sentara.com

Matthew M. Murawski, R.Ph., Ph.D.
Associate Professor of Pharmacy Administration
Department of Pharmacy Practice
Purdue University
West Lafayette, Indiana
murawski@pharmacy.purdue.edu

Agatha L. Nolen, MS, D.Ph., FASHP
Director, OPPS
HCA—Regulatory Compliance Support
Nashville, Tennessee
agatha08@comcast.net

John M. Petrich, R.Ph., MS
Clinical Manager
Investigational Drug Service
Cleveland Clinic
Cleveland, Ohio
PETRICJ@ccf.org

Jerry Robinson, Pharm.D.
Clinical Specialist, Surgical—Trauma ICU
Chairperson, Medication Safety Committee
Department of Pharmacy
Huntsville Hospital
Huntsville, Alabama
jerry010@hhsys.org

Gisela I. Robles, Pharm.D.
Assistant Professor
College of Pharmacy
Nova Southeastern University
Clinical Pharmacy Coordinator at Coral Springs Medical Center
Fort Lauderdale, Florida
rgisela@nova.edu

Pazit Shaked, Pharm.D., BCPS
Geriatrics Ambulatory Service Clinical Specialist
Shosh District
Israel
shpazitsh@clalit.org.il

Susan J. Skledar, R.Ph., MPH
Associate Professor, School of Pharmacy
University of Pittsburgh
Director, Drug Use and Disease Management Program and Investigational Drug Service
University of Pittsburgh Medical Center
Department of Pharmacy & Therapeutics
Pittsburgh, Pennsylvania
SkledarSJ@upmc.edu

Linda S. Tyler, Pharm.D., FASHP
Director, Drug Information Service
University of Utah Hospitals & Clinics
Salt Lake City, Utah
Linda.Tyler@hsc.utah.edu

Angela R. Vinti, Pharm.D., BCPS
Assistant Clinical Professor of Pharmacy Practice
Auburn University Harrison School of Pharmacy
Mobile Satellite Campus
Adjunct Assistant Professor of Family Medicine
University of South Alabama
Mobile, Alabama
arv0001@auburn.edu

Frank Vitale, MA
National Director
Pharmacy Partnership for Tobacco Cessation
University of Pittsburgh School of Pharmacy
Pittsburgh, Pennsylvania
vitalef@pitt.edu

Meghan F. Wilkosz, Pharm.D.
Clinical Pharmacy Specialist—Acute Medicine
Adjunct Clinical Instructor
University of Connecticut School of Pharmacy
VA Connecticut Healthcare System Pharmacy Service
West Haven, Connecticut
Meghan.wilkosz@va.gov

Alan J. Zillich, Pharm.D.
Research Scientist
Center for Excellence in Implementing Evidence-Based Practices
Roudebush VA Medical Center
Assistant Professor
School of Pharmacy and Pharmaceutical Sciences
Purdue University
West Lafayette, Indiana
azillich@purdue.edu

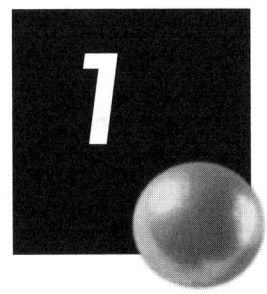

A Multidisciplinary Approach to Venous Thromboembolism Prophylaxis in a Community Hospital

Jered B. Bauer

Background and Introduction

Venous Thromboembolism (VTE), which includes deep vein thrombosis (DVT) and pulmonary embolism (PE), is recognized as the most preventable cause of inpatient mortality.[1] Retrospective analysis has indicated PE is associated with 10% of all inpatient mortality.[2] With the potential for nine out of 10 DVTs to go undiagnosed,[3] VTE has the characteristics of a silent killer. The DVT Free Registry that enrolled 5,451 hospitalized patients with documented DVT revealed that only 29% of all patients had received prior prophylaxis within 30 days of DVT diagnosis.[4] Of those without prior prophylaxis, 59% were nonsurgical, medically ill patients.[4] These findings from the DVT Free Registry illustrate the need for routine VTE risk assessment and prophylaxis in the inpatient setting.

Beginning in 2005, The Joint Commission™ and National Quality Forum (NQF) began working together to establish standards of care relating to prevention and treatment of DVT.[5] It is more apparent each passing day that to satisfy potential future standards and pay-for-performance criteria, healthcare institutions will need to demonstrate that routine measures are in place not only for identifying patients at risk for VTE, but also for improving VTE outcomes.* Improving patient care within an institution can be a daunting task. Many variables may limit success. A multidisciplinary approach is often required for achievement of hospital-wide initiatives. VTE risk assessment and prophylaxis is one such hospital-wide initiative that needed to be addressed at St. Elizabeth's Hospital.

Description of the Multidisciplinary Approach

St. Elizabeth's Hospital is a 506-bed, licensed community facility located in Belleville, Illinois. Inpatient admissions exceed 13,000 annually, with an additional 160,000 outpatient visits each year.[6] Over 40 medical specialties are represented by physician staff. To initiate focus on VTE at St. Elizabeth's Hospital, pharmacy leadership developed a comprehensive VTE risk assessment and prophylaxis order form (see Figure 1.1). This form was presented to the pharmacy and therapeutics (P&T) committee during a July 2005 meeting. P&T reviewed the form during a presentation from

---

*Over the past 2 years, the focus within development of the National Consensus Standards for the Prevention and Care of Deep Vein Thrombosis has been narrowed to specifically address issues surrounding surgical risk of VTE.

Venous Thromboembolism (VTE) Prophylaxis

Complete this VTE risk assessment upon admission for all patients. Guidelines for VTE prophylaxis focus upon group-specific patient risk factors taking into account medical history, clinical signs, and existing condition. Prophylaxis selection should be determined from the assessed patients cumulative risk score.
These guidelines reflect current recommendations supported by clinical evidence, but do not supersede clinical judgment. These recommendations do not apply to all patients in all clinical situations. The patients risk status may change requiring reassessment.

VTE Prophylaxis Orders (Check all that apply):

Early mobilization (check one): ☐Assist to ambulate   or   ☐PT referral for ambulation
☐Graduated compression stocking: ☐Knee high (will be used if nothing specified)   or   ☐Thigh high
☐Calf pneumatic compression device (if contraindication to calf device, utilize foot pneumatic compression device)
☐Heparin 5,000 units SC (check one):   ☐q 8 hr   or   ☐q 12 hr
☐LMWH: _____
☐Warfarin: _____
☐Other: _____
No prophylaxis needed (check one):   ☐Not indicated   or   ☐Contraindicated   or   ☐Currently in place

Physician Signature: _____ **Date:** _____

Total Risk Factor Score	Incidence of DVT	Risk Level	Prophylaxis Regimen
0–1 Points	<10%	Low risk	No specific measures; early and aggressive ambulation
2 Points	10–20%	Moderate risk	LDUH q 12 hr, GCS, or IPC
3–4 Points	20–40%	High risk	LDUH q 8 hr, or IPC
≥5 Points	40–80%	Highest risk	LMWH, Warfarin (INR 2–3), or IPC/GCS + LDUH q 8 hr

IPC=intermittent pneumatic compression   GCS=graduated compression stockings   LDUH=low-dose unfractionated heparin   LMWH=low molecular weight heparin

Risk Assessment (Check all that apply and add together for total risk score) Risk Score = _____

1 POINT FOR EACH RISK FACTOR	2 POINTS FOR EACH RISK FACTOR	3 POINTS FOR EACH RISK FACTOR	5 POINTS FOR EACH RISK FACTOR
☐Age 40 to 60 years ☐CHF, myocardial infarction ☐Estrogen therapy or OCs ☐Inflammatory bowel disease ☐Major surgery planned or within past month ☐Minor surgery (<1 hr duration) ☐Obesity (BMI >30) ☐Pregnancy, postpartum (<1 month) ☐Varicose veins, peripheral edema	☐Central venous catheterization ☐Immobility, bed rest >24 hr ☐Age >60 ☐Nephrotic syndrome ☐COPD, acute respiratory failure, pneumonia ☐Major surgery (>1 hr duration)	☐Malignancy, chemotherapy ☐Mechanical ventilation ☐Hx of DVT, PE or (Fam Hx) ☐Hypercoaguable state Activated protein C resistance (Factor V Leiden) Antithrombin III deficiency Protein C or S deficiency Prothrombin gene mutation Hyperhomocysteinemia Antiphospholipid antibodies Other	☐CVA/paralysis (5) ☐Total knee arthoplasty (5) ☐Spinal cord injury (5) ☐Total hip arthoplasty (5) ☐Pelvis/hip/leg fracture, major trauma (5)

Absolute Contraindications	Relative Contraindications
☐Active bleeding ☐Warfarin in pregnancy ☐Uncontrolled HTN ☐Intraocular, CNS injury ☐Epidural, indwelling spinal catheter ☐Head, spine, or extremity trauma without hemostasis ☐Allergies to heparin or enoxaparin ☐Thrombocytopenia (platelet count <100K) ☐History of heparin induced thrombocytopenia	☐Proliferative retinopathy ☐Spinal catheter/tap ☐CNS neoplasm ☐Prior CNS, GI, or GU bleed ☐Recent (<24 hr) epidural catheter ☐Concomitant antiplatelet agents, NSAIDs, or other anticoagulant agents in patients at increased risk of hemorrhage

Recommendations:
- For planned manipulation of an epidural or spinal catheter (insertion, removal), LMWHs should be avoided/held for 24 hr before manipulation, then resumed no earlier than 2 hr following manipulation.
- For heparin/LMWH therapy, monitor CBC daily; for warfarin therapy, monitor PT/INR.

St. Elizabeth's Hospital
211 South Third Street
Belleville, IL 62220

Figure 1.1. Original VTE Assessment and Prophylaxis Order Form (reprinted with permission from St. Elizabeth's Hospital, Belleville, IL).

pharmacy, approved it, and adopted VTE prophylaxis as an institution-wide performance improvement initiative. Additionally, P&T formed a multidisciplinary VTE group. The VTE group was an ad hoc committee comprised of pharmacy (chair), nursing, and medical staff; information technology (IT); and risk management members. P&T requested the VTE group to review the institution's current VTE prophylaxis practice and identify opportunities for improvement. The VTE group needed a total of two meetings to assess the institution's VTE prophylaxis practices and develop an outline of the best approach to improving them.

Baseline data gathered for the group to review included pharmacologic VTE prophylaxis rates. VTE prophylaxis rates were determined through a review of hospital statistics from the month of August 2005. Specifically, hospital statistics showed a total of 5,496 total inpatient days for the month. Review of the same month revealed that only 808 (14.7%) total inpatient days were administered pharmacologic VTE prophylaxis. Vascular lab data revealed that approximately 1 in every 88 discharges (1.13%) suffered an ultrasound-confirmed DVT as an inpatient. Information was also requested from Health Information Services (HIS) to determine the number of ICD-9-CM coded discharges for embolism (see Table 1.1).

The HIS report indicated a 1.1% rate of discharge-diagnosed VTE. This rate seemed low to the VTE group. After all, it was lower than the statistics provided from the vascular lab. The rates reported by HIS were dependent upon proper documentation of VTE within the patient's chart. The VTE group theorized the low rates were due to a lack of VTE awareness among practitioners. The group thought it was possible to not only improve prophylaxis and decrease VTE rates, but also to increase awareness (and, consequently, revenue through more accurate documentation and discharge diagnosis coding). Attempting to improve identified practices and patient outcomes, the VTE group decided the best approach to reach these goals was through electronic patient risk assessment.

The VTE group decided to include an electronic assessment of patient risk factors for VTE upon admission. This approach seemed most practical, since nursing already performed detailed electronic admission assessments that often revealed many of the defined VTE risk factors, such as those identified through past medical history (e.g., prior thrombosis), admitting diagnosis (e.g., spinal injury), and physical exam (e.g., obesity). The VTE group reviewed the American College of Chest Physicians (ACCP) 7th conference guideline for the prevention of DVT.[7] Risk factors for VTE were extracted from this reference and assigned scores (see Figure 1.2). Patient VTE risk levels, including low, moderate, high, and highest risk based upon populations and total risk factor scores,

Table 1.1. ICD-9-CM Discharge Diagnosis Reviewed

ICD-9-CM Code Reviewed	Description
415.1	Pulmonary embolism and infarction
415.11	Iatrogenic pulmonary embolism and infarction
453.4	Venous embolism and thrombosis of deep vessels of lower extremity
435.41	Venous embolism and thrombosis of deep vessels of proximal lower extremity
453.42	Venous embolism and thrombosis of deep vessels of distal lower extremity
453.8	Venous embolism and thrombosis of other specified veins
453.9	Venous embolism and thrombosis of unspecified veins

Patient:		Age:	Location:	MD:

Risk: ☐ <10% (0–1 pt.),   ☐ 10–20% (2 pt.),   ☐ 20–40% (3–4 pt.),   ☐ 40–80% (≥5 pt.)

Risk Factors: <u>1 pt.</u>:☐ Age 40–60;☐ Systolic HF/MI; ☐ Estrogen tx; ☐ Obesity; ☐ IBD; ☐ Surgery < 1hr
            <u>2 pt.</u>: ☐ Age >60; ☐ Immobility/bed rest >24 hr;
                ☐ Major surgery >1 hr; ☐ Pulmonary disease
            <u>3 pt.</u>: ☐ Cancer; ☐ Mechanical ventilation; ☐ History of DVT/PE or hypercoagulable state
            <u>5 pt.</u>: ☐ CVA/Paralysis; ☐ Spinal injury; ☐ Knee/hip replacement;
                ☐ Pelvic/hip/leg fracture/trauma

Contraindications to Anticoagulation: ☐ YES: _____ ☐ NO

Recommendation: ☐ Heparin 5,000 units q 8 h, ☐ Enoxaparin 30 or 40 mg q 24 h (circle dose), ☐SCDs

Recommendation Accepted: ☐ YES ☐ NO Date: _____   Rx initiated (if different): _____

- -
<u>30-Day Followup:</u>
   VTE: ☐ YES ☐ NO Date: _____   Mortality: ☐ YES ☐ NO Date : _____
   Readmission: ☐ YES ☐ NO Date: _____   Bleeding: ☐ YES ☐ NO Event:_____

Figure 1.2. VTE Tracking Form.

were developed. When electronic assessment was performed, it would risk stratify patients into the VTE risk groups of low, moderate, high, or highest risk groups. Once the patient was identified as being part of a particular VTE risk category, a care plan specific to each group would be generated by the clinical computer system. Care plans could include orders for mechanical prophylaxis, ambulation, and alerts to physicians about the need for VTE prophylaxis. To risk stratify the patient the clinical computer system had to be capable of tabulating total weighted scores for all identified risk factors. Additionally, to close the gap on overlooked patients, a daily report would generate in the pharmacy including all moderate to highest risk patients admitted in the prior 24 hours without VTE prophylaxis. Pharmacy would then review each patient for contraindications to prophylaxis and contact the primary physician with a recommendation for VTE prophylaxis. Although it was clear to the group this was the best approach, a significant technological obstacle existed with this plan: IT determined the current clinical computer system was not able to incorporate risk scoring. Therefore, it would be impossible to electronically stratify patients into low, moderate, high, or highest risk categories. Addressing this obstacle would require nursing to duplicate parts of their admission assessment (e.g., by charting in the clinical computer system and reiterating similar information on a written form), tabulating total risk score, and initiating care plans based upon risk stratification. Consequently, the VTE group decided implementing this strategy would place too much additional strain on nursing's already significant workload.

The group then focused its efforts back on the manual VTE form that had been presented to P&T. At the request of the committee's physician members, the form's layout was revised to optimize legibility and ease of use. The VTE assessment and prophylaxis form was added to the electronic records system so that it printed automatically for all new admissions. The admitting nurse placed the VTE form in the front of each patient's chart to be completed by the treating physician.

The institution also emphasized the necessity of educating hospital staff, physicians, and patients to increase VTE awareness. Prior to implementing use of the form upon patient admission, the VTE group intensively educated the hospital staff and physicians about this initiative. Educational endeavors included drafting a "Dear Doctor" letter (detailing program information and VTE statistics) that was mailed to all physicians on staff. Posters were created through the hospital's marketing department to increase VTE awareness and encourage prophylaxis. Posters were placed in all patient care areas and in all physician lounges. Presentations were developed addressing VTE statistics and detailing the elements of appropriate VTE risk assessment and prophylaxis. These presentations were given to medical staff at executive meetings, nursing through inservices, and administrative staff. Additional information was delivered to hospital and medical staff via pharmacy and medical staff newsletters. The VTE group also developed a patient education flyer through the marketing department to increase VTE awareness among patients.

Results of the Multidisciplinary Approach

Three months into using the form on all new admissions, performance measures, including VTE rates and patient days with prophylaxis, were reviewed and compared to baseline measures. The results revealed underutilization of the VTE form with only minimal improvement in VTE prophylaxis rates (see Table 1.2) and prompted the group to discuss further options. The VTE group was at a loss for ways to improve hospital practices regarding VTE assessment and prophylaxis. However, pharmacy leadership identified an opportunity to stimulate hospital-wide improvement and offered to develop a pharmacist-led program to assess all new admissions for risk of VTE and recommend appropriate pharmacologic prophylaxis. The VTE group was unanimous in support for this approach.

To assist the pharmacist in identifying patients at risk of VTE, IT developed a daily report including all new admissions within the past 24-hour period. Another report was developed by IT to include all patients actively receiving heparin or low molecular weight heparin (LMWH). Each morning the pharmacist cross-referenced the admissions with the patients receiving heparin or LMWH to identify patients requiring an assessment. To facilitate physician approval of recommendations and to create a manageable program, only patients identified to be either high or highest risk would have recommendations made and placed into their charts. Additionally, maternity, nursery, pediatric, and psychiatry patients would be excluded from the program.

The VTE risk assessment and prophylaxis form proved useful as an aid in development of the pharmacist-led program. The form was broken down into two parts. The first part became a tracking sheet that included risk assessment and could be used to follow up on recommendations made (see Figure 1.2). The second part was a bold 3" x 5" sticker that would include the identified risk factors, incidence of VTE, and specific recommendation for prophylaxis (see Figure 1.3). The sticker would be placed directly in the progress notes of the patient's chart for the physician to review and either sign into an order or deny the recommendation. Once all patients were assessed and recommenda-

Table 1.2. VTE Risk Assessment and Prophylaxis Form Program

Measure	Baseline (August 2005)	Post-VTE Form 3 Month Review (June 2006)
Total of Patient Days	5,493	5,065
Total Days of Pharmacologic VTE Prophylaxis	808	912
Patient Days with VTE Prophylaxis	14.7%	18.0%
Inpatient Diagnosed Ultrasound Confirmed DVT	1.1%	1.1%

ATTENTION PHYSICIAN

This patient is at ☐ HIGH (20–40%)　　☐ HIGHEST (40–80%) risk for VTE

Identifiable risk factors include

☐ Age >40	☐ Surgery
☐ Systolic HF, MI	☐ Pulmonary disease
☐ Obesity (≥30% IBW)	☐ Cancer
☐ Immobility >24 hr	☐ Mechanical ventilation
☐ History of DVT/PE	☐ Knee or hip replacement
☐ CVA or paralysis	☐ Pelvic, leg, or hip fracture or major trauma

Other: _____

If patient does not have contraindications to anticoagulation, please consider prophylaxis with
　　☐ Heparin 5,000 units q 8 hr
　　☐ Enoxaparin 40 mg q 24 hr
　　☐ Enoxaparin 30 mg q 24 hr (Est. CrCl <30 mL/min)
　　☐ Patient is at risk but has contraindications for anticoagulation; recommend mechanical prophylaxis

---

Figure 1.3. VTE Recommendation Sticker.

tions placed in the respective charts the pharmacist reviewed the tracking sheets from the previous 4 days for accepted recommendations.

Pharmacy also provided quarterly reviews to P&T to mark program progress. Measures reviewed include percent patient days receiving VTE prophylaxis (total days of VTE prophylaxis for the month were provided from the heparin and LMWH reports and were divided by total inpatient days for the month) and inpatient diagnosed VTE rates via daily reports from the vascular lab. Two quarterly performance reviews have been completed since implementation of the pharmacist-led VTE program. The first review revealed a 103% improvement in patient days with pharmacologic VTE prophylaxis from 14.7% to 30.7%. Vascular lab data revealed a four-fold reduction in in-patient-diagnosed DVT rates from one in every 88 discharges to one in every 422 discharges. In the second review (6 months into the program) patient days with VTE prophylaxis had improved 209% over baseline and DVT rates maintained greater than a four-fold reduction (see Table 1.3). Cumulative tracking of recommendations made since inception of this program reveal an average of 58 accepted recommendations out of 193 made per month.

To justify increased costs in the pharmaceutical budget incurred from use of this program, cost-savings were assigned to each accepted recommendation. To determine cost savings a number needed to treat of 10 patients to prevent one VTE[8] was chosen with an average cost savings of $10,000[9] assigned to each inpatient VTE prevented. This model generated a cost savings of $1,000 for each accepted recommendation. All savings assignments were based on evidence throughout the medical literature that have revealed additional healthcare costs associated with treatment of inpatient diagnosed VTE. Considering that recommendations within this program are made only on high to highest risk patients this cost-saving estimation is conservative. Using this model the pharmacist-led VTE prophylaxis program has provided the institution an estimated cost-saving benefit of approximately $450,000 over 7 months.

Table 1.3. Pharmacist-Led VTE Risk Assessment and Prophylaxis Program

Measure	Baseline (August 2005)	R.Ph. VTE Program 3 Month Review (March 2007)	R.Ph. VTE Program 6 Month Review (June 2007)
Total of Patient Days	5,493	5,629	5,100
Total Days of Pharmacologic VTE Prophylaxis	808	1,750	2,333
Patient Days with VTE Prophylaxis	14.7%	31.1%	45.7%
Inpatient Diagnosed Doppler Confirmed DVT	1.1% (1 in 88 discharges)	0.2% (1 in 422 discharges)	0.1% (1 in 1,177 discharges)

Conclusion

A pharmacist-led VTE prophylaxis program was not the VTE group's first approach to improving VTE prophylaxis rates at St. Elizabeth's. However, given the limitations encountered, the group ultimately came up with a successful plan to improve VTE risk assessment and prophylaxis for St. Elizabeth's Hospital. This initiative has provided a tremendous benefit for the institution through improved patient outcomes, increased VTE awareness, and overall decreased expenses. Success with this multidisciplinary effort has further recognized the pharmacist as an essential part of the patient care team within the hospital setting.

References

1. Gross P, Weitz JI. Increasing awareness, optimizing prevention, and advancing treatment for VTE. American Society of Hematology. Available at: http://www.hematology.org/publications/hematologist/JA07/practicing.cfm#A. Accessed September 10, 2007.
2. Sandler DA, Martin JF. Autopsy proven pulmonary embolism in hospital patients: are we detecting enough deep vein thrombosis? *J R Soc Med.* 1989;82(4):203-205.
3. Hirsh J, Hoak J. Management of deep vein thrombosis and pulmonary embolism a statement for healthcare professionals from the council on thrombosis (in consultation with the council on cardiovascular radiology), American Heart Association. *Circulation.* 1996;93:2212-2245.
4. Goldhaber SZ, Tapson VF. A prospective registry of 5,451 patients with ultrasound-confirmed deep vein thrombosis. *Am J Cardiol.* 2004;93:259-262.
5. National Quality Forum: National Consensus Standards for the Prevention and Care of Venous Thromboembolism (including Deep Vein Thrombosis and Pulmonary Embolism). Available at: http://www.qualityforum.org/projects/ongoing/vte/index.asp. Accessed August 20, 2007.
6. http://www.steliz.org/about/facts_and_statistics.php.
7. Geerts WH, Pineo GF, Heit JA, et al. Prevention of venous thromboembolism: the seventh ACCP conference on antithrombotic and thrombolytic therapy. *Chest.* 2004;126(suppl);338s-400s.

8. Samama MM, Cohen AT, Darmon JY, et al. A comparison of enoxaparin with placebo for the prevention of venous thromboembolism in acutely ill medical patients (MEDENOX). *N Engl J Med.* 1999;341:793-800.

9. MacDougall DA, Feliu AL, Boccuzzi SJ, et al. Economic burden of deep-vein thrombosis, pulmonary embolism, and post-thrombotic syndrome. *Am J Health Syst Pharm.* 2006;63(suppl): S5-S15.

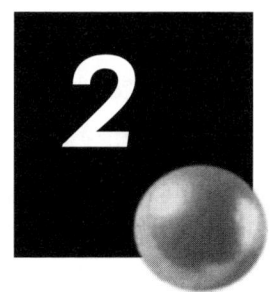

FMEA or FEMA: Preventing Your Next Anticoagulation Disaster Using Existing Failure Mode Effects Analysis

Linda S. Tyler

Acknowledgments: The author would like to recognize the contributions and support of the Utah Patient Safety Steering Committee—Adverse Drug Event Users Group, and the University of Utah Hospitals & Clinics FMEA anticoagulation teams.

The Federal Emergency Management Agency (FEMA) and failure mode effects analysis (FMEA) sound similar, are both in some way related to disasters, and both help protect lives. However, the similarity ends there. FEMA is called in when there is a huge disaster, such as Hurricane Katrina. In healthcare, when there is a medication error, it often feels like a huge disaster, but unfortunately FEMA does not help in this kind of disaster.

Overview

FMEA is a technique used in many industries to analyze processes, identify ways to improve processes and sources of failure, and ultimately to prevent harm. FMEA can be applied to many healthcare processes.[1-3] The steps in performing an FMEA are as follows:

- Create a flowchart of the current process—both a high level and detailed flowchart (Figures 2.1 and 2.2)
- Identify steps in the process where the process may fail (Figure 2.2)
- Analyze the causes and effect of failure (Figure 2.3)
- Score the analysis considering likelihood an effect would occur, severity of event if it occurred, and the ability to detect the event. Several methods exist to score an FMEA.[1,3] One method is presented in Table 2.1. The purpose of the scoring is to assist in identifying and prioritizing those steps that pose the highest vulnerability for causing failure.
- Summarize analysis by identifying steps in the process most likely to fail and cause harm (Figure 2.4)
- Identify potential actions to prevent harm or improve the process (Figure 2.5)
- Prioritize those actions
- Rescore to assess the improvement (if desired)

High Level Flowchart

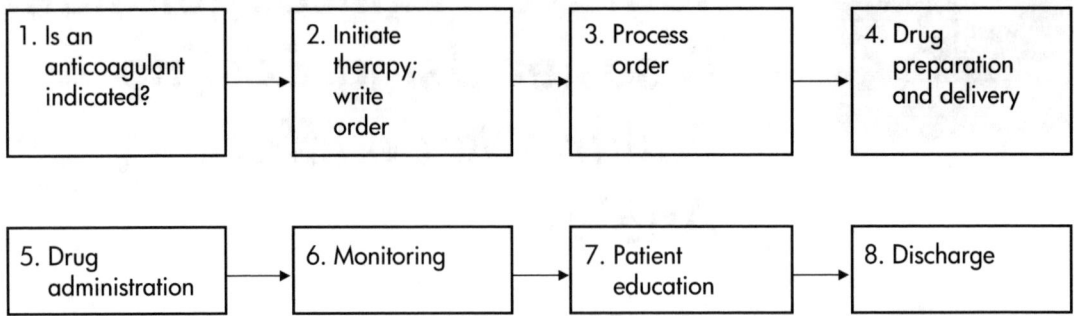

Figure 2.1. High Level Flowchart of Steps in the Medication-Use Process for Use of Anticoagulants.

Source: From the Utah Patient Safety Steering Committee, Adverse Drug Effects User Group. Failure Mode Effects Analysis on High Risk Drugs: Anticoagulant Agents for Inpatient Use. January 2005. Available at: www.uha-utah.org. Used with permission.

Detailed Flowchart

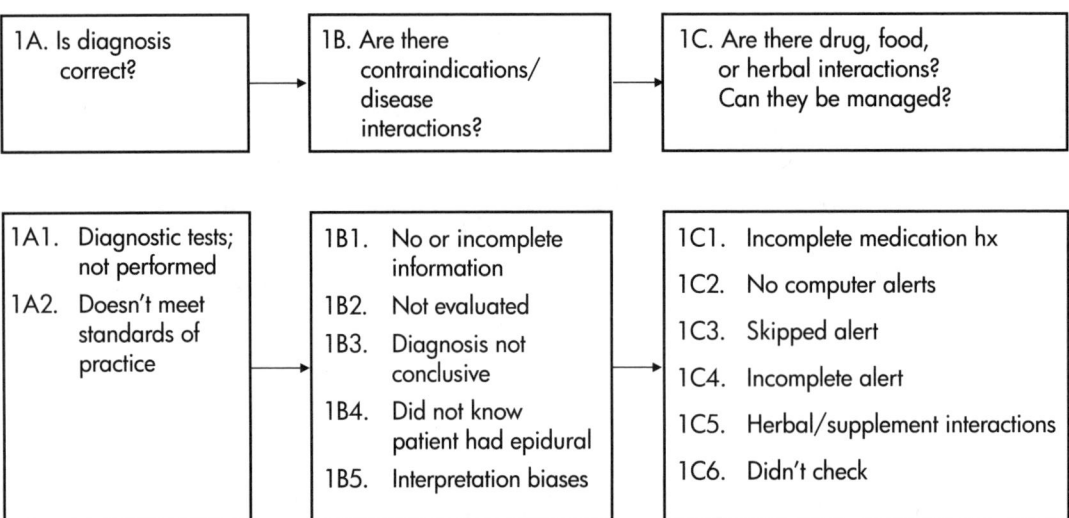

Figure 2.2. Detailed Flowchart and Failure Modes for Each Step Using the First Step in Figure 2.1 as an Example.

Source: From the Utah Patient Safety Steering Committee, Adverse Drug Effects User Group. Failure Mode Effects Analysis on High Risk Drugs: Anticoagulant Agents for Inpatient Use. January 2005. Available at: www.uha-utah.org. Used with permission.

The "Pearl"

So here is the Pearl: Use existing FMEA projects and adapt them to your organization to save a significant amount of time and energy. You can use existing FMEAs to identify potential areas for improvement for your organization. These FMEAs can also provide the framework for projects **specific to your organization.** At a minimum, you can look at the results from other organizations and see if they offer opportunities for you to improve care in your institution.

Assess Failure Causes and Effects

- ☐ 1. Is anticoagulant indicated?
- ☐ 1A. Is diagnosis correct?
- ☐ Failure causes
  - ■ Diagnostic tests not performed
  - ■ Doesn't meet standard of practice
- ☐ Failure effects
  - ■ Anticoagulant administered when not indicated
  - ■ No treatment when indicated
  - ■ Failure of diagnostic test
  - ■ Inappropriate prescribing

Figure 2.3. Assess Failure Causes and Effects—Example of First Step from Detailed Flowchart in Figure 2.2.

Source: From the Utah Patient Safety Steering Committee, Adverse Drug Effects User Group. Failure Mode Effects Analysis on High Risk Drugs: Anticoagulant Agents for Inpatient Use. January 2005. Available at: www.uha-utah.org. Used with permission.

Table 2.1. Scoring an FMEA[a]

Scoring Item	Range of Values	Score Interpretation
Likelihood	1–10	1 = not likely to occur 10 = very likely to occur
Severity	1–10	1 = very unlikely harm will occur 10 = very likely that severe harm will occur
Likelihood of detection	1–10	1 = very likely to be detected 10 = very unlikely to be detected
Risk priority number (RPN)	1–1,000	Multiply likelihood, severity, and likelihood of detection score

[a]Institute for Healthcare Improvement FMEA tool.[1]

Sources of Existing FMEAs

FMEA projects can be obtained from several sources. If you are searching for examples online, be sure to search for both *FMEA* as well as *healthcare failure mode effects analysis* (HFMEA) as results might be found under either term. Currently, there are not any good medical subject headings (MeSH) to identify this technique in PubMed. Several sources regularly have information on FMEA[1-4]: The Institute for Healthcare Improvement (IHI) (www.ihi.org),[1] Institute for Safe Medication Practices (ISMP) (www.ismp.org),[2] and the Veterans' Administration National Center for Patient Safety (NCPS) (www.patientsafety.gov).[3,4] IHI has many examples of specific FMEA projects, many of them related to medication use issues.[5] In addition, the Utah Hospital Association has recently made available the FMEA project that was conducted on anticoagulants.[6] Utah implemented Patient Safety Regulations in 2001. To help support patient safety initiatives, the Utah Patient Safety Steering Committee (UPSSC) was formed. This committee is a collaboration of the Utah Department of Health, the Utah Hospital Association, and HealthInsight, the peer-review organization for Utah

High Vulnerabilities in Using Anticoagulants

The following steps in the process were identified as being vulnerable to failure for many organizations.

- Checking for contraindications to anticoagulants
- Checking for drug and food interactions
- Double-checking preparation in the pharmacy
- Drug available from floor stock
- Nursing override of anticoagulant medication orders and administering prior to a pharmacist's check of the order
- Failure to monitor patient and check for signs of bleeding and thrombotic disease progression
- Failure to educate patients and their caregivers about their underlying disease state, how to use their medication, and what to do in the event of an adverse drug reaction
- Duration of therapy not clearly established when patient starts receiving these medications
- Followup appointments not established for patient
- Followup with primary care provider does not occur
- Patient unable to attend followup appointment
- Patients do not get prescriptions filled or have gaps in their therapy

Figure 2.4. High Vulnerabilities in Using Anticoagulants.

Source: From the Utah Patient Safety Steering Committee, Adverse Drug Effects User Group. Failure Mode Effects Analysis on High Risk Drugs: Anticoagulant Agents for Inpatient Use. January 2005. Available at: www.uha-utah.org. Used with permission.

Actions to Reduce Occurrence of Failure from Anticoagulants

Several consistent themes emerged from the process as ways to prevent failure in the system. These are summarized below.

- Establish and follow guidelines and protocols for the indications, dosing, and monitoring of anticoagulant therapy. Developing and following standard practices and following can reduce the risk of failure in many parts of the process. A bibliography of current literature guidelines and examples from several hospitals are included in the appendices. The appendices also include Web resources available on this topic, many including current guidelines and methods to implement them.
- Consider anticoagulants other than heparin when appropriate. Heparin presents more opportunities for medication errors because of its availability in many different concentrations, various modes of preparation, and that it may be used by several different routes of administration.
- Assign clear accountabilities for monitoring such as checking the laboratory values and adjusting the dose as necessary.
- Develop alerting systems to notify clinicians of abnormal laboratory values.
- Use standard concentrations for parenteral anticoagulants.
- Consider the use of "smart" pumps or other safety checks to prevent infusion related medication errors.
- Develop a standard process for educating patients and their caregivers on the underlying disease, how to take their medication, and what to do in the event of an adverse event.
- Assign clear accountabilities for patient education.
- Establish a standard process with clear accountabilities for the continuity of patient care after discharge including set followup appointment, establish who will provide ongoing care for anticoagulant therapy, communicate with primary care giver, and address barriers to obtaining prescriptions and getting to followup appointments.
- Double-check therapy at transfer of care situations.

Figure 2.5. Actions to Reduce Occurrence of Failure from Anticoagulants.

Source: From the Utah Patient Safety Steering Committee, Adverse Drug Effects User Group. Failure Mode Effects Analysis on High Risk Drugs: Anticoagulant Agents for Inpatient Use. January 2005. Available at: www.uha-utah.org. Used with permission.

and Nevada. A subcommittee of this group is the Adverse Drug Event Users Group (ADEUG). One of the projects this group conducted was an FMEA on anticoagulants. These materials are available on the Utah Hospital Association Web site, www.uha-utah.org, under publications. The Utah project used the IHI methodology for preparing and scoring the project. This methodology was considered easier to work with from a "just in time" training perspective. Participants could be trained in how to use the tool within a few minutes. This training ease was important for the Adverse Drug Event Users Group, since not everyone could attend every meeting and new members joined the group throughout the project.

High-risk drugs lend themselves well to an FMEA approach, as well as to using existing FMEAs and applying them to your organization. The reason FMEAs work well for high-risk drugs is that the risk of these medications is the same everywhere. With anticoagulants, for instance, the consequences of an overdose would be a severe bleed and potentially death. The risk of too low a dose would be the development of thrombosis and death. These risks are universal. Likewise, the drug use process will have similar elements in every organization. Every pharmacy will have to procure and store the drug, order it, prepare and dispense it, administer it, and monitor the effect of the therapy. Figure 2.1 can easily be adapted to any high-risk drug as a high-level flowchart.

Using an Existing FMEA

Here is an example of how the anticoagulant FMEA from the Utah project can be applied to your organization:

Begin by reading the FMEA's executive summary. This executive summary lists high vulnerabilities (Figure 2.4) and actions to reduce failure (Figure 2.5). You can review these vulnerabilities and actions and see if any of them apply to your organization. Do you have opportunities to improve in any of these areas?

A second way to use existing FMEAs is as an example of how FMEAs are put together. If you have never done an FMEA it can be pretty daunting. Once you can see some examples, it becomes much easier. You can then conduct your own FMEA on a topic relevant to your organization.

Another way is to use existing FMEAs as a "skeleton" for your own project. You can gather a team to conduct an FMEA. The team can review the flowcharts, the failure mode effects analysis, and the effects of failure. These can then be adapted to your organization to make them useful and relevant. Then you can conduct the scoring specific to your organization. Based on the scoring, you can identify your high priority areas. When you have a framework such as this, a project that may take ordinarily 20–30 hours can be reduced to 2–4 hours. It can typically be very time-consuming to create the flowcharts and spreadsheets with the failure modes, effects, and scoring. It is sometimes hard to get physicians and other staff to participate in the flowcharting and "nitty-gritty" failure mode effects analysis. However, it may be reasonable to have them spend a couple of hours reviewing existing materials and giving their impression of the risks of a particular problem in your institution. A reason to not use an existing FMEA as a framework would be if the FMEA seems to have more differences than similarities to your organization.

Many projects available on the Web, such as the Utah project, provide materials (such as spreadsheets and flowcharts) in formats that you can easily adapt and use your own institution's scoring. When using another organization's project, you can compare your scoring to that organization. Doing so offers you the opportunity to see if your results make sense in comparison.

Some of the key "take homes" (Figure 2.5) from the Utah project can be applied to many organizations in several different ways. While this FMEA evaluated anticoagulants, the lessons are equally relevant to other high-risk drugs.

• Use standardized protocols and preprinted orders. Doing so will help reduce the chances of harm for any high-risk drug. Using standard, evidence-based processes helps reduce chances of error.

- Assign clear accountability for all steps in the medication use and monitoring process. For instance, it is often unclear who should check the lab values or alerts, or who is responsible for conducting patient education and making followup appointments.

- Decrease use of heparin. A controversial recommendation of the anticoagulant FMEA was to reduce the use of heparin. As team members conducted the analyses, it was clear that heparin added more harm to the medication use and monitoring process than other alternatives. For instance, heparin comes in many different concentrations and, consequently, increases opportunities for storage and preparation errors. In contrast, enoxaparin comes in a prefilled syringe in a set concentration. Further, since heparin is often given as an infusion, it is easy to see how it poses more risk from a system analysis perspective. Heparin is also more likely to cause heparin-induced thrombopenia than low molecular weight heparins. A companion recommendation was to use "smart" pumps or other double checks to reduce the chance of administration errors.

- Use a standard process for educating patients. This recommendation was viewed as essential to prevent harm for patients that leave the hospital on anticoagulants. It is important for the patient or his/her caregiver to be clear on how to use their medication, how to prevent medication-related harm, and the plan for followup care and appointments. Also, anticoagulant patients should know their INR goal and the likely duration of therapy.

- Use double checks at transfer of care situations. This recommendation is critical to prevent inadvertent dosage changes or the medication not administered.

The University of Utah Hospitals & Clinics applied a statewide FMEA project to the organization. Task team members were asked to commit 2 hours to a meeting, then 30 minutes reviewing materials after the meeting. The task team included seven pharmacists (representing drug information, medical/surgical units, ambulatory care, and anticoagulation specialists), five nurses (representing risk management, quality improvement, and medical surgical units), and seven physicians (the medical director, hospitalists, and representatives from pulmonary, medicine, laboratory, and hematology). One-fourth of those participating were also members of the pharmacy and therapeutics (P&T) committee. Medicine and pharmacy residents were also included in the process. The 2-hour meeting included reviewing the statewide project (20 minutes), dividing into groups of three to four (five groups total) and scoring two pages of the FMEA specific to the University of Utah Hospitals & Clinics (45 minutes). The group updated the spreadsheet (10 minutes) and reviewed the results (20 minutes). The team identified key vulnerabilities within the institution and then developed key areas to be addressed, based on the scoring priorities (25 minutes). University of Utah Hospitals & Clinics scoring priorities were similar to the statewide scoring (Table 2.1) with a couple of differences. In comparing the University of Utah Hospitals & Clinics' results with the statewide scores, the University of Utah Hospitals & Clinics scored lower for administration because the institution uses "smart pumps" but scored higher on the patient education items and the continuity of care from inpatient to outpatient. The summary was written up, reviewed by the team, then presented to the P&T committee. Of the eight action items developed by the team, the P&T committee selected two to work on first. Work on the other action items continued over the next year. The team thought this approach was very successful, as most of the team's time was spent working on the action items, rather than in the initial set up of the project.

Summary

In summary, FMEA is a useful technique to analyze processes and to identify the steps that could fail and potentially produce harm. There are many resources available to guide you through an FMEA as well as many examples of existing FMEAs. Using existing FMEAs can save you valuable time and help you identify risk points faster. FMEAs are rewarding projects since they offer the opportunity to proactively prevent harm.

References

1. Institute for Healthcare Improvement. Failure Mode Effects Analysis Tools. Available at: http://www.ihi.org/ihi/workspace/tools/fmea/. Accessed September 4, 2007.

2. Institute for Safe Medication Practices. Failure Mode and Effects Analysis: A tool to help guide error prevention efforts. Available at: http://www.ismp.org/Tools/FMEA.asp. Accessed September 4, 2007.

3. United States Department of Veterans Affairs, National Center for Patient Safety. Using Healthcare Failure Mode Effects Analysis. Available at: http://www.va.gov/ncps/SafetyTopics/HFMEA/HFMEA_JQI.html. Accessed September 4, 2007.

4. United States Department of Veterans Affairs, National Center for Patient Safety. HFMEA cognitive aid. Available at: http://www.va.gov/ncps/CogAids/HFMEA/index.html. Accessed September 4, 2007.

5. Institute for Healthcare Improvement. All FMEA Tools. Available at: http://www.ihi.org/ihi/workspace/tools/fmea/AllTools.aspx. Accessed September 4, 2007.

6. Utah Patient Safety Steering Committee, Adverse Drug Effects User Group. Failure Mode Effects Analysis on High Risk Drugs: Anticoagulant Agents for Inpatient Use. January 2005. Available at: www.uha-utah.org.

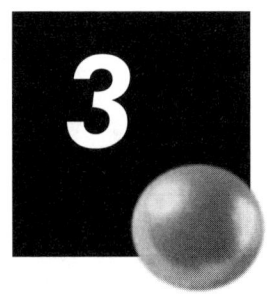

The Heparin Protocol: If It Can Be Done Wrong, It Will Be

Sharon R. Baty

Michele Durda

Jerry Robinson

Unfractionated heparin is included on the Institute for Safe Medication Practices (ISMP) list of high-alert medications due to its potential to cause serious adverse effects. In addition, complicated therapeutic regimens requiring frequent monitoring and dose adjustments make heparin administration risky. For this reason, an 800-bed community hospital has focused considerable efforts on improving the safety and quality of the IV heparin therapy protocol process.

Background

In the winter of 2004, the hospital implemented a revised IV heparin therapy protocol. The previous approach of "one dose fits all" was no longer the standard of care. Specifically, initial heparin dosing recommendations varied based on the disease state being treated so the IV heparin therapy protocol was revised. Ironically, the quest to improve the protocol resulted in a big problem. Heparin protocol related medication error reports increased from baseline by approximately three to five reports per month!

Let's start from the beginning. The original IV heparin therapy protocol was developed in the 1990s and consisted of an initial bolus dose of 80 units/kg and an initial infusion rate of 16 units/kg/hr. Heparin protocol medication usage evaluations (MUEs) were completed annually from 1999 to 2003 and revealed compliance with the protocol was low. However, the MUE results showed when used correctly, the protocol usually resulted in therapeutic PTT values. In an effort to increase compliance, heparin protocol education was completed by the pharmacy department. The education included presentations to the nursing units that most frequently used the heparin protocol. Flyers were also displayed throughout the hospital. Correct protocol usage increased immediately following intensive education; however, over time compliance with the protocol would again decrease.

In 2003, the hospital's cardiology pharmacy & therapeutics (P&T) committee recommended revising the protocol. The American College of Cardiology/American Heart Association 1999 acute myocardial infarction guidelines and 2002 unstable angina and non-ST-segment elevation myocardial infarction guidelines contained heparin-dosing recommendations. Based on these guidelines, the cardiology P&T committee approved a *cardiology* regimen consisting of an initial bolus dose of 60 units/kg and initial infusion rate of 12 units/kg/hr. Simultaneously, the hospital's stroke committee approved a *stroke/TIA/no bolus* regimen consisting of no initial bolus and initial infusion rate of 16 units/kg/hr.

After multiple revisions and numerous committee reviews, the revised IV heparin therapy protocol was implemented in the winter of 2004 (see Figure 3.1). The final version contained three initial regimens (general, cardiology, and stroke/TIA/no bolus) and three sliding scale regimens

IV Heparin Therapy Protocol 2004

Revised 1/13/04

DATE	IV HEPARIN THERAPY PROTOCOL:
	1. Obtain baseline PTT and CBC (if not done in last 48 hr).
	2. Calculate patient's weight in kg (_____ lb ÷ 2.2 = _____ kg)
	3. Select General, Cardiology, or Acute Stroke/TIA/No Bolus heparin regimen. Initial bolus, initial infusion rate, and sliding scale regimen (high, standard, or low) must be indicated by physician. If not specified, contact physician. Use drip strength of heparin 25,000 units/250 mL D_5W (100 units/mL) unless ordered otherwise. Use calculations below only when using standard drip 100 units/mL. For loading dose and drip rate round off to nearest 100 units.
	☐ General
	Loading dose of 80 units/kg (80 units x _____ kg = loading dose). Maximum loading dose is 10,000 units.
	Start heparin drip at 16 units/kg/hr immediately after bolus. Drip rate in mL/hr = (16 units x _____ kg) ÷100.
	Maximum initial drip rate 1,500 units/hr.
	☐ Cardiology
	Loading dose of 60 units/kg (60 units x _____ kg = loading dose). Maximum loading dose is 5,000 units.
	Start heparin drip at 12 units/kg/hr immediately after bolus. Drip rate in mL/hr = (12 units x _____ kg) ÷ 100.
	Maximum initial drip rate 1,000 units/hr.
	☐ Acute Stroke/TIA/No Bolus
	No loading dose unless otherwise specified. Start heparin drip at 16 units/kg/hr.
	Drip rate in mL/hr = (16 units x _____ kg) ÷ 100. Maximum initial drip rate 1500 units/hr.
	4. STAT PTT 6 hr after heparin has been started and then q AM.
	5. Sliding Scale Regimen
	Based on results of PTT, adjust heparin as follows using regimen specified by MD. If sliding scale not specified, contact physician. For Acute Stroke/TIA/No Bolus regimen, give NO bolus doses unless otherwise specified.

IF PTT:	_____ HIGH	_____ STANDARD	_____ LOW
<50	5,000 units bolus—increase by 200 units/hr	3,000 units bolus—increase by 200 units/hr	3,000 units bolus—increase by 200 units/hr
50–70	3,000 units bolus—increase by 200 units/hr	2,000 units bolus—increase by 100 units/hr	NO CHANGE
71–91	1,000 units bolus—increase by 100 units/hr	NO CHANGE	NO CHANGE
92–114	NO CHANGE	NO CHANGE	Hold x 1 hr
115–143	NO CHANGE	Decrease by 100 units/hr	Hold x 1 hr—decrease by 100 units/hr
144–182	Decrease by 200 units/hr	Decrease by 200 units/hr	Hold x 1 hr—decrease by 200 units/hr
>182	Hold x 1 hr—decrease by 200 units/hr	Hold x 1 hr—decrease by 200 units/hr	Hold x 1 hr—decrease by 200 units/hr

	6. If PTT >182 or <50, repeat PTT 2 hr after heparin dose adjusted.
	7. Call physician if PTT >182 or <50 on two consecutive samples.
	8. Repeat PTT 6 hr after dosage change and adjust per above sliding scale.
	9. When PTT is in desired range with no dosage change necessary, PTT should be drawn q AM only.
	10. RN to write any change in heparin dosage on heparin sticker and place on physician's order sheet.
	11. Platelet count q 3 d.
	Physician's signature:

Place patient label in this box

Place stat label in this box

Date: _____

Time: _____

Room No. _____

Figure 3.1. Original 2004 IV Heparin Therapy Protocol Order Set.

(high, standard, and low). Prescribers were asked to specify the initial starting regimen and sliding scale when the protocol was ordered. This specification reflected a change from the original protocol. Previously, prescribers ordered *heparin protocol* because there was only one initial regimen and if not specified, the standard sliding scale served as the default. Another change that affected nursing and the laboratory department was the timing of PTT values. In the revised protocol, PTT values were to be ordered 6 hours after initiation of the infusion and 6 hours following subsequent dosage adjustments. In the original protocol, PTT values were ordered 8 hours after initiation and subsequent adjustments.

One additional change included a heparin sticker pilot project on a few high-use nursing units (see Figure 3.2). Previous MUEs had demonstrated various violations including incorrect bolus doses, drip rate adjustment errors, and inappropriate timing of PTT samples. With the original protocol, the nursing staff had to write orders in the chart each time a heparin protocol adjustment was made. The orders often did not contain all pertinent information. A multidisciplinary group, comprised of various hospital personnel, recommended standardizing this process by using preprinted heparin stickers with blanks for the PTT result, heparin bolus (if indicated), heparin rate adjustments, and timing for the next PTT. For heparin rate adjustments, the stickers would be completed and placed in the order section of the chart.

Housewide education about the new heparin protocol was completed by the pharmacy department along with the hospital's education council, a committee comprised of nurse educators and representatives from the hospital's major clinical departments, prior to implementation. Numerous educational tools were utilized including an article in the hospital newsletter, presentations to multidisciplinary service lines, distribution of flyers throughout the hospital, and presentations at nursing and pharmacy staff meetings. Unfortunately, Murphy's law of medication use prevailed: "If it can be done wrong, it will be; if a work-around exists, it will be used."

During the summer of 2004, an MUE concluded that correct heparin protocol usage had declined. Protocol violations included regimen (initial or sliding scale) not specified in the initial order, incorrect initial bolus and/or drip rate, incorrect adjustments, and inappropriate timing of PTT samples. Staff education was again recommended and completed. The MUE indicated the use of the heparin stickers resulted in fewer adjustment errors so this pilot project was expanded housewide. As seen with previous MUEs, correct usage of the protocol usually resulted in therapeutic PTT values.

In the following spring of 2005, another MUE was completed that showed correct protocol usage had declined further. Protocol violations occurred throughout the medication-use process. Staff education was recommended, but clearly, as seen in the previous heparin MUEs, education alone was unlikely to resolve the problem. The MUE results were presented to the medication safety committee because of concerns about the increased heparin protocol related medication error reports.

Heparin Adjustment Sticker

PTT (time) results _____ (_____)
Heparin bolus (if indicated) _____units
Hold heparin (if indicated) _____
Increase/Decrease heparin drip rate by _____units/hr to
_____ units/hr or _____ mL/hr
Next PTT due at _____
Signature _____

Figure 3.2. Heparin Adjustment Sticker (printed on 1″ by 4″ adhesive labels).

Heparin Safety Committee Activities

After identifying and evaluating the errors associated with the application of the IV heparin therapy protocol, the medication safety committee focused on finding solutions for the problem. The recommendation of the committee was to create another committee to tackle the "heparin issue," and a heparin safety committee was born.

Heparin Safety Committee Composition

The medication safety pharmacist (pharmacy department) and the patient safety coordinator (quality management department) were appointed as chairs of the brand new committee. Members were selected from volunteers representing numerous departments, including nurse educators from the surgical and medical service lines, and clinical pharmacy specialists from the cardiac areas and the surgical trauma intensive care unit. Because the identified problems were associated with accurately carrying out the hospital's standard protocol, rather than the appropriateness of the protocol itself, the committee decided to focus on the implementation of the heparin protocol after the order was written. To facilitate understanding about the practical problems associated with using the heparin protocol on a daily basis on the nursing units, a charge nurse involved in daily patient care on a cardiac unit with high utilization of the heparin protocol and a unit secretary were recruited to join the committee.

Evaluating the Heparin Protocol Process

The first meeting of the heparin safety committee occurred in August of 2005. The first action of the committee was to break down the heparin protocol process into individual steps in an attempt to identify potential weaknesses. The committee identified eight discrete steps in the initiation of the heparin protocol and seven steps for any necessary dose adjustments.

Heparin Protocol Process-Initiation

1. Prescriber orders "heparin per protocol" (telephone order, written order, or written order on preprinted protocol order set).
2. Baseline PTT performed.
3. Nurse clarifies the specific protocol regimen and sliding scale with the prescriber as necessary.
4. Nurse completes the heparin protocol order set as necessary.
5. Heparin protocol is entered into the computer system by the unit secretary.
6. Pharmacist reviews orders.
7. Heparin is administered.
   a. Bolus dose (if required) is double-checked by a second nurse.
   b. Infusion rate is double-checked by a second nurse.
8. PTT is checked 6 hours after heparin initiated.

Heparin Protocol Process-Adjustment

1. Out-of-range PTT result is identified.
2. Information is recorded on heparin sticker (new infusion rate, if bolus or hold required, next PTT), and the sticker is placed in the Physician's Order Section of the patient's chart.

3. New infusion rate and bolus dose (if required) entered into the computer system by the unit secretary.

4. Pharmacist reviews orders.

5. Heparin is adjusted.

   a. Bolus dose (if required) is double-checked by a second nurse.

   b. Infusion rate is double-checked by a second nurse.

6. Repeat PTT 2 hours after heparin dose adjusted if PTT >182 seconds or <50 seconds. Repeat PTT 6 hours after heparin dose adjusted for all other PTT values.

7. When PTT is in desired range with no dosage change necessary, PTT is drawn once every morning only.

Some of the problems identified by the committee in the existing process included issues with the prescriber not specifying an initial regimen or sliding scale for dose adjustments, incorrect dose adjustments, doses administered prior to pharmacist review, followup PTTs not entered or scheduled for the wrong time, and inconsistency in the documentation of dose adjustments. To alleviate some of these issues, the committee considered the following changes:

1. Reformat heparin protocol order set to be more readable and "less busy."

2. Implement a heparin flowchart on the back of the heparin protocol to replace the stickers and require the documentation of all PTT values, including therapeutic values.

3. Improve the format of the heparin protocol order set and documentation in the computer system, for implementation with the new electronic medical record and computer system (anticipated completion date, 2008).

4. Provide education to staff on the number and types of errors occurring with the heparin protocol.

The committee assigned several committee members to prepare a draft of the reformatted heparin protocol and flowchart for presentation at the following meeting.

The Updated Protocol and Flowchart and Housewide Implementation

One of the problems identified by the heparin safety committee involved the actual protocol order sheet. When the sheet was originally developed, the purpose was to cover every point and leave nothing to interpretation. The actual sheet layout included so much information that the sheet was difficult to follow.

The order sheet was edited more for layout than content. Although changes had occurred with different doses and interval of next followup PTT, the overall instructions remained unchanged. The first thing that occurred with editing was removal of unnecessary page lines that were a part of the original document. The next major adjustment was making the initial bolus and rate more easily visible. Although originally each protocol (general, cardiology, and stroke) had its own bolus and initial drip rate specifications with empty lines to complete, the team felt that a single box with the necessary information would be easier to read and follow. A reminder statement to contact the physician if the initial regimen or sliding scale regimen were not specified in the order was also added to the form. The statement not to give bolus doses with acute stroke/TIA regimens was kept in a similar position but was made more prominent with the other changes in the document. After numerous modifications suggested by multiple professionals seeing the revisions, the heparin safety committee approved the document at the September 2005 meeting for use in a 1-month pilot (see Figure 3.3). Additionally, the team chose to print the document on yellow paper for quick identification in the medical record.

The development of the heparin flowchart (see Figure 3.4) for documentation also helped with several problem areas identified by the heparin safety committee. The heparin flowchart incorporated the information on the previously used heparin sticker, but also provided for documentation of the independent double check by a second nurse and for transcription documentation. This flowchart was eventually printed on the back of the heparin order sheet so that both documents were in the same chart location. The unit secretaries were instructed to avoid removing these protocols from thinned charts until the protocol was complete. Printing the protocols on yellow paper also helped identify the orders in the written medical chart. A few months later, a problem was identified where nurses were using the wrong protocol after a protocol was changed from a *standard* to a *low* or *high* sliding scale. To help identify completed heparin order sheets, bright pink stickers were designed to show that the heparin protocol had been changed or was no longer in effect.

After having all aspects of the form updated, the new protocol order sheets and corresponding flowcharts were implemented on three nursing areas for a 1-month pilot during October 2005 based on recommendations from the hospital's medication safety committee. At the conclusion of the pilot, audits and surveys were completed to identify problems and obtain feedback on using the updated sheets and procedures. The 1-month pilot was considered a success because no heparin protocol related medication errors were reported on the pilot units during the month of October. In addition, the new protocol format and flowchart were well-received by both nursing and medical staff based on written comment forms and verbal surveys at staff meetings. Small changes were made to the protocol format and flowchart based on feedback from the pilot nursing units. The finalized documents were approved by the hospital's medication safety committee and quality council, with the recommendation to adopt the new process throughout the hospital. A start date in February 2006 was selected and a coordinated housewide education campaign was organized prior to the roll-out. The medication safety pharmacist updated pharmacists on the new protocol. Nurses were informed through staff meetings and printed posters placed in every nursing area prior to housewide implementation. Unit secretaries were inserviced about the new protocol at their regular staff meetings. Physicians were notified through articles in the P&T newsletter.

Measuring Success

In spring 2006, a heparin MUE was completed to assess whether protocol compliance improved. Correct protocol usage had increased by 33% from the MUE completed the previous year! The protocol was specified by prescribers in all reviewed cases except one. There was also only one initial bolus and drip rate violation. The majority of violations were adjustment or monitoring violations, but the number of these violations had decreased overall. The reformatted protocol along with the implementation of the heparin flowchart was working!

When developing and implementing a complex protocol or procedure, the most important aspect is to continue monitoring success and failures, and to adapt the protocol to the changing healthcare system. Also, a fresh prospective can be very beneficial. In the case of the heparin protocol, the new medication safety pharmacist brought in ideas that had not been previously recognized at the institution. A pharmacist who specialized in cardiology also noticed a dosing change that was needed to comply with current guidelines. A centralized medication occurrence reporting system allowed for identification of reported problems, which were assessed, resulting in process changes

Physician's Orders

Document in patient record
Critical value addressed per protocol

Revised 1/06 jlr

ADULT IV HEPARIN THERAPY PROTOCOL:

1. Obtain baseline PTT and CBC (if not done in last 48 hr).

2. Calculate patient's weight in kg: _____ lb ÷ 2.2 = _____ kg

3. Physician must specify regimen (General, Cardiology, or Acute Stroke/TIA/No Bolus) AND sliding scale adjustment desired (High, Standard, or Low). If not specified, contact physician.

☐ GENERAL	☐ CARDIOLOGY	☐ ACUTE STROKE/TIA/No Bolus
Loading dose: 80 units/kg (Maximum 10,000 units)	Loading dose: 60 units/kg (Maximum 5,000 units)	Loading dose: None
Infusion: 16 units/kg/hr (Maximum 1,500 units/hr or 15 mL/hr)	Infusion: 12 units/kg/hr (Maximum 1,000 units/hr or 10 mL/hr)	Infusion: 16 units/kg/hr (Maximum 1,500 units/hr or 15 mL/hr)

Loading Dose: _____ units x _____ kg = _____ units IVP (round to nearest 100 units)

Infusion (25,000 units/250 mL D5W): _____ units x _____ kg/100 = _____ mL/hr (round to nearest mL/hr)

4. Stat PTT 6 hr after heparin has been started and then q AM. Adjust per sliding scale.
5. RN to record all PTT values and heparin dose changes on heparin flowchart (see reverse).
6. Platelet count q 3 d.
7. Sliding Scale Regimen

Adjust heparin using regimen specified by MD.
For Acute Stroke/TIA/No Bolus regimen, give NO bolus doses unless otherwise specified.

IF PTT:	☐ HIGH	☐ STANDARD	☐ LOW
<50	5,000 units bolus—increase by 200 units/hr	3,000 units bolus—increase by 200 units/hr	3,000 units bolus—increase by 200 units/hr
50–70	3,000 units bolus—increase by 200 units/hr	2,000 units bolus—increase by 100 units/hr	NO CHANGE
71–91	1,000 units bolus—increase by 100 units/hr	NO CHANGE	NO CHANGE
92–114	NO CHANGE	NO CHANGE	Hold x 1 hr
115–143	NO CHANGE	Decrease by 100 units/hr	Hold x 1 hr—decrease by 100 units/hr
144–182	Decrease by 200 units/hr	Decrease by 200 units/hr	Hold x 1 hr—decrease by 200 units/hr
>182	Hold x 1 hr—decrease by 200 units/hr	Hold x 1 hr—decrease by 200 units/hr	Hold x 1 hr—decrease by 200 units/hr

8. Repeat PTT 6 hr after dosage change (unless PTT >182 or <50, see #9 below).
9. If the PTT is >182 or <50, repeat PTT 2 hr after heparin dose adjustment.
10. Call physician if PTT >182 or <50 on two consecutive samples.
11. When PTT is in desired range with no dosage change necessary, PTT should be drawn q AM only.

Physician's signature: _____

Place patient label in this box

Date: _____

Time: _____

Figure 3.3. Revised IV Heparin Therapy Protocol Order Set.

Heparin Drip Adjustment Flowchart

Heparin drip started at (date and time) _____

1. PTT Date:_____ Time:_____
   PTT results _____
   ☐ No Change. Continue heparin drip at _____ mL/hr.
   ☐ Heparin bolus (if indicated) _____ units
   ☐ Hold heparin (if indicated) _____ hr
   ☐ Increase/decrease heparin drip rate by _____
       units/hr to _____ units/hr or _____mL/hr.
   ☐ Next PTT due at Date: _____Time: _____
   Signature   Cosign
	2. PTT Date:_____ Time:_____
	   PTT results _____
	   ☐ No Change. Continue heparin drip at _____ mL/hr.
	   ☐ Heparin bolus (if indicated) _____ units
	   ☐ Hold heparin (if indicated) _____ hr
	   ☐ Increase/decrease heparin drip rate by _____
	       units/hr to _____ units/hr or _____mL/hr.
	   ☐ Next PTT due at Date: _____Time: _____
	   Signature Cosign

HUC[a]:	HUC[a]:

3. PTT Date:_____ Time:_____
   PTT results _____
   ☐ No Change. Continue heparin drip at _____ mL/hr.
   ☐ Heparin bolus (if indicated) _____ units
   ☐ Hold heparin (if indicated) _____ hr
   ☐ Increase/decrease heparin drip rate by _____
       units/hr to _____ units/hr or _____mL/hr.
   ☐ Next PTT due at Date: _____Time: _____
   Signature   Cosign
	4. PTT Date:_____ Time:_____
	   PTT results _____
	   ☐ No Change. Continue heparin drip at _____ mL/hr.
	   ☐ Heparin bolus (if indicated) _____ units
	   ☐ Hold heparin (if indicated) _____ hr
	   ☐ Increase/decrease heparin drip rate by _____
	       units/hr to _____ units/hr or _____mL/hr.
	   ☐ Next PTT due at Date: _____Time: _____
	   Signature Cosign

HUC[a]:	HUC[a]:

5. PTT Date:_____ Time:_____
   PTT results _____
   ☐ No Change. Continue heparin drip at _____ mL/hr.
   ☐ Heparin bolus (if indicated) _____ units
   ☐ Hold heparin (if indicated) _____ hr
   ☐ Increase/decrease heparin drip rate by _____
       units/hr to _____ units/hr or _____mL/hr.
   ☐ Next PTT due at Date: _____Time: _____
   Signature   Cosign
	6. PTT Date:_____ Time:_____
	   PTT results _____
	   ☐ No Change. Continue heparin drip at _____ mL/hr.
	   ☐ Heparin bolus (if indicated) _____ units
	   ☐ Hold heparin (if indicated) _____ hr
	   ☐ Increase/decrease heparin drip rate by _____
	       units/hr to _____ units/hr or _____mL/hr.
	   ☐ Next PTT due at Date: _____Time: _____
	   Signature Cosign

HUC[a]:	HUC[a]:

7. PTT Date:_____ Time:_____
   PTT results _____
   ☐ No Change. Continue heparin drip at _____ mL/hr.
   ☐ Heparin bolus (if indicated) _____ units
   ☐ Hold heparin (if indicated) _____ hr
   ☐ Increase/decrease heparin drip rate by _____
       units/hr to _____ units/hr or _____mL/hr.
   ☐ Next PTT due at Date: _____Time: _____
   Signature   Cosign
	8. PTT Date:_____ Time:_____
	   PTT results _____
	   ☐ No Change. Continue heparin drip at _____ mL/hr.
	   ☐ Heparin bolus (if indicated) _____ units
	   ☐ Hold heparin (if indicated) _____ hr
	   ☐ Increase/decrease heparin drip rate by _____
	       units/hr to _____ units/hr or _____mL/hr.
	   ☐ Next PTT due at Date: _____Time: _____
	   Signature Cosign

HUC[a]:	HUC[a]:

Patient label here
	9. PTT Date:_____ Time:_____
	   PTT results _____
	   ☐ No Change. Continue heparin drip at _____ mL/hr.
	   ☐ Heparin bolus (if indicated) _____ units
	   ☐ Hold heparin (if indicated) _____ hr
	   ☐ Increase/decrease heparin drip rate by _____
	       units/hr to _____ units/hr or _____mL/hr.
	   ☐ Next PTT due at Date: _____Time: _____
	   Signature Cosign

[a]Health Unit Coordinator

Figure 3.4. Heparin Drip Adjustment Flowchart.

during the implementation process. Lastly, methods that work for one protocol may or may not work for other protocols. However, the heparin flowchart concept has since been adapted to monitor glucose values and insulin infusion changes for the hospital's insulin infusion protocols.

Looking back at the planning and implementation of the IV heparin therapy protocol improvement process, the heparin safety committee identified several keys to the success of the project. These fundamental concepts will be utilized during future safety and quality initiatives.

Keys to Success

- Multidisciplinary participation—particularly involvement of a motivated frontline nurse and a unit secretary
- Small scale pilot on three nursing units identified kinks before housewide implementation
- Coordinated educational efforts in advance of roll-out—education provided to nursing staff through flyers and nurse staff meetings, education provided to unit secretaries through unit secretary staff meetings, and education provided to pharmacists through pharmacy staff meetings

Future Plans

Although significant improvement in the use of the IV heparin therapy protocol was measured following the implementation of the revised protocol and flowchart, the medication safety and heparin safety committee members recognize that there is still room for enhancement. The pharmacy department is continuing to monitor the use of the IV heparin therapy protocol through annual medication-use evaluations to ensure that the gains are maintained. In addition, with the announcement of the new 2008 Joint Commission™ National Patient Safety Goal on anticoagulants, a new anticoagulant safety group is being planned. The new group will continue to focus on the safe use of heparin. One of the areas targeted for improvement is the format of the IV heparin therapy protocol in the hospital's computer system. The anticoagulant safety group will take an active role in the development of the heparin therapy order set in the upcoming medical information system (to be implemented 2008) and automated alert screening. The medication safety committee anticipates continued success with the multidisciplinary approach to medication safety initiatives and further improvements in the use of the IV heparin therapy protocol.

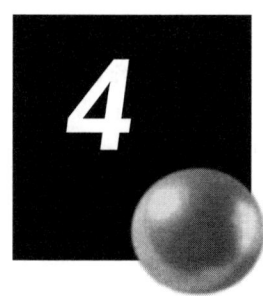

STEMI and Trauma—One and the Same

Sandra L. Chase
Kathleen Johnston

Abstract

A comprehensive, quality improvement initiative at Spectrum Health (a community-based academic health system privately owned with multiple provider groups and inpatient facilities) in Grand Rapids, Michigan has improved the standard of care for acute myocardial infarction (AMI) patients with ST-segment elevation (STEMI). The effort, which began in 2003, has decreased the time from arrival in the emergency department (ED) to reperfusion of the myocardium in the catheterization laboratory (Cath Lab) to a median of 64 minutes—well below the national standard of 90 minutes. The Grand Rapids AMI Quality Team designed a unique STEMI alert process—similar to a trauma code—which clearly defines the responsibilities of all team members, minimizes opportunities for error, decreases precatheterization preparation time, and streamlines the decision-making process.

Introduction

In most patients presenting with acute myocardial infarction with ST-segment elevation, or STEMI, rapid percutaneous coronary intervention (PCI) is the preferred method to reperfuse the myocardium. Because early use of angioplasty has been shown to reduce mortality and morbidity and preserve cardiac muscle viability, the Joint Commission™ has set a standard of 90 minutes from ED arrival to primary PCI for STEMI patients (Joint Commission Standards, www.hms.gov).

Studies have shown that historically, hospitals have had significant opportunity for improvement in meeting this arrival-to-PCI goal. One study published in 2006 consisting of 33,647 patients in 421 hospitals from 1999 to 2002 shows that less than 35% of patients received primary PCI within the 90-minute standard.[1]

The American College of Cardiology has created an initiative supported by more than 20 national professional societies called "D2B [door-to-balloon]: An Alliance for Quality," which was launched to help healthcare organizations overcome the challenges of meeting this primary PCI standard. The D2B Alliance acknowledges that, "Accomplishing this level of performance can be an organizational challenge."[2]

A literature study conducted by the D2B Alliance found strong evidence for three major strategies in meeting and exceeding this measure—activation of the Cath Lab using emergency medicine physicians rather than cardiologists, effective use of prehospital EKGs, and monitoring of performance data and providing feedback based on that monitoring.[3]

These proven strategies and several others have been employed at Spectrum Health—a community-based, privately owned, not-for-profit health system with multiple provider groups in western Michigan with seven hospitals and more than 140 service sites. At Spectrum Health hospitals in Grand Rapids, a multidisciplinary team set out to streamline ED and Cath Lab systems to ensure that patients receive PCI within 90 minutes of arrival in the ED as measured by median time to balloon inflation and attainment of the 90-minute target 100% of the time.

Methods

The Grand Rapids Acute Myocardial Infarction (AMI) Quality Team has primary responsibility for the time-to-PCI improvements. A quality improvement specialist from the Spectrum Health Quality Department was responsible for bringing together all of the disciplines that needed to be involved to improve time to PCI for STEMI patients. The approximately 25-member team is interdisciplinary and interdepartmental. Members of the team include ED physicians, cardiologists, hospitalists, physician executives, nurse executives, nurse managers, pharmacy staff, clinical nurse specialists, dietary personnel, care managers, the director of cardiovascular services, a Cath Lab nurse manager, a quality improvement specialist, a research database coordinator, a manager of coding operations and bed management; and nurses from the ED, Cath Lab, and floor.

Early on in the improvement initiative, two nationally recognized cardiology experts in angioplasty and STEMI treatment were brought in to engage in group discussions with Spectrum Health physicians about the importance of reducing the time from arrival to PCI for these patients. These discussions helped to convince physicians that meeting this goal was a necessity, not an option.

Strong physician and clinical leads championed the improvement efforts from the beginning. This created close collaboration among ED and cardiology physicians. Team leadership was shared among the ED, cardiology, and the quality department. The team began developing the process by researching best practice and taking a detailed look at each step of the process as it was currently being carried out. Gaps between best practice and current process were identified and discussed, looking for opportunities for improvement. To accomplish this process, a data collection method was developed in which each component of the process was timed.

The ED recorded times for the following:

- Onset of cardiopulmonary symptoms
- Patient arrival at the ED
- First EKG
- Patient evaluated by ED physician
- Cardiologist paged
- Cardiologist responded
- Cath Lab team activated
- Cath Lab team ready
- Patient left ED

The Cath Lab recorded the following times:

- Patient arrived in Cath Lab (table time)
- Physician arrival
- First wire across lesion
- First balloon inflation

Data were recorded on "orange sheets," easily recognized by their color (Figure 4.1). The process data on each STEMI patient were then taken to monthly AMI quality team meetings and analyzed. The team looked for acceptable reasons for delays, and recommended solutions for tightening the process where possible. Control charts, which showed the monthly data of the component steps, were developed and shared with physicians and members of the multidisciplinary team in all areas (see results). This led to many improvements in the process and streamlining of care.

The team developed a STEMI alert process similar to a trauma code, which emphasized the urgency of caring for the STEMI patient and initiated an identified chain of actions. Key to this process was the development of a STEMI alert packet, initiated in the ED, which included appropriate order sets, the "orange sheets" for recording each step of the process, an acute coronary syndrome information sheet, physician order sheets for the ED and hospital nursing units, and checklists for the physician, nurse and secretary with identified job accountabilities. This process was very helpful for several reasons: 1) it helped to clarify the role of each team member; 2) it standardized the team's response by line-listing each element of individual roles, so the process could proceed without having to rely on memory; and 3) it included tools, such as the "orange sheet" that was readily available to collect data on the STEMI alert process.

It is essential in process improvement that data are current and reflect nearly real-time performance. Usually data are compiled for each patient progressing through the STEMI process within one business day of treatment. A clinical decision support analyst from the quality department completes any outstanding data elements on the "orange sheets." Immediate feedback to providers and the team can be provided and issues can be resolved in "near real time," when issues are recent and memorable. The director of cardiology sends letters to the physicians who do not comply with one of the Joint Commission standards including, no angiotensin converting enzyme inhibitor (ACEI)/angiotensin receptor blocker (ARB), no aspirin (ASA), no beta blocker, and no cardiology discharge instructions (Table 4.1). An example of the "No ASA" letter is included as Figure 4.2.

By breaking the process into small steps, it has been easier for the team to see any delays in the process. It became evident very early in the work that the process was not really linear; in fact, multiple steps could and should occur simultaneously. The practitioners doing the work—in the ED, the Interventionalist's practice, and the Cath Lab—made process improvements in each setting.

Internally the data were shared at meetings, on flyers posted on quality bulletin boards, and posted on the Spectrum Health Web site. Progress was recognized within the quality team, and in meetings of executives and the board. Externally, the organization has marketed the door-to-PCI times in billboard and advertising campaigns. Celebrating the team's successes periodically has helped to spread pride in the members' work and rewards the unending effort of the team.

As the process improvement matured and many of the easier improvements ("low-hanging fruit") were made, the group began to look for other strategies that could be used to speed time to treatment. The team began to explore having the ED physician activate the Cath Lab. Initially, there was concern that the ED physician might call in the interventionalist inappropriately. This concern

ED Copy
Time Study for STEMI Alerts
STAYS IN ED

Cerner Sticker

Date	ED Physician:	Phone #
Patient Name	Cardiologist:	
Patient MR #	ED Charge Nurse Phone # 14999	
ED Nurse	ED Secretary	

INDICATOR		TIME
Time of Onset of CP Symptoms		
Time Patient Arrived ED		
Time of 1st EKG		*(Circle one)* Pre-Hospital Hospital
Time Patient Evaluated by ED Physician		
Time Cardiologist Paged	ED Completes	
Time Cardiologist Responded		
ED Physician activate Cath Lab? Y N (circle one)		
Time Cath Lab Team Activated		
Time Cath Lab Team Ready		
Time Patient Left ED		
Time Patient Arrived in Cath Lab Room (Table Time)		
Physician Arrival	Cath Lab Completes	
Lido Time		
Access Time		
Time of 1st Wire across Lesion		
Time to TIMI 3 Flow		
Time of 1st Balloon Inflation		

THIS FORM TO STAY IN THE ED IN DEDICATED SLOT. DO NOT SEND WITH PATIENT TO FLOOR

Comments / Suggestions:

NOT PART OF THE MEDICAL RECORD

Figure 4.1. Orange Sheet.

Table 4.1. Joint Commission Standards for Acute Myocardial Infarction (AMI)

ID#	Name	Description	Type of Measure	Age Groups
AMI-1	Aspirin at arrival	AMI patients without aspirin contraindications who received aspirin within 24 hours before or after hospital arrival	Process	18 and older
AMI-2	Aspirin prescribed at discharge	AMI patients without aspirin contraindications who are prescribed aspirin at hospital discharge	Process	18 and older
AMI-3	ACEI or ARB for LVSD	AMI patients with left ventricular systolic dysfunction (LVSD) and without ACE inhibitor (ACEI) or ARB contraindications who are prescribed an ACEI or ARB at discharge	Process	18 and older
AMI-4	Adult smoking cessation advice/counseling	AMI patients with a history of smoking cigarettes, who are given smoking cessation advice or counseling during the hospital stay	Process	18 and older
AMI-5	Beta blocker (BB) prescribed at discharge	AMI patients without beta blocker contraindications who are prescribed a beta blocker at hospital discharge	Process	18 and older
AMI-6	Beta blocker (BB) at arrival	AMI patients without beta blocker contraindications who received a beta blocker within 24 hours after hospital arrival	Process	18 and older
AMI-7	Time to thrombolysis	Median time from arrival to administration of thrombolytic agent in patients with ST segment elevation or LBBB on the ECG performed closest to the hospital arrival time	Process	18 and older
AMI-8	Time to PTCA	Median time from arrival to PTCA in patients with ST segment elevation or LBBB on the ECG performed closest to hospital arrival time	Process	18 and older
AMI-9	Inpatient mortality	AMI patients who expired during hospital stay	Outcome	18 and older

March 10, 2006
Source: National Hospital Core Measures and the Joint Commission.

did not materialize. In the very rare event that the interventionalist was called in inappropriately, the case was reviewed and followup was initiated. The obvious advantage to this new process was that ED physicians were able to activate the Cath Lab at the same time they contacted the cardiologist. There was no delay in waiting for the cardiologist to arrive and review the EKG and then to finally call in the catheterization team and wait for their arrival.

Another strategy that was instrumental in improving time to treatment for STEMI patients was limiting all cardiology calls to cardiology interventionalists. Instead of having a noninterventionalist initiate treatment and subsequently discover the need to call in an interventionalist, STEMI calls

NO ASA

Date: _____

To: _____, MD
Address

Re: Patient Name:
    Medical Record #:
    Discharge Date:

Dear_____:

We appreciate the efforts that you've made in improving quality care with myocardial infarction patients at Spectrum Health. As part of our ongoing review, we note that the patient did not have documentation for why they were not discharged on aspirin.

The Joint Commission™ requires AMI patients who are not discharged on aspirin to have clear documentation of the reason why. Although we realize it is extra effort, we would very much appreciate your help in complying with these Joint Commission mandates and specifically state the contraindication for aspirin.

Thank you again for your efforts in regards to good quality care for our acute myocardial patients.

Sincerely,

Director of Cardiology, MD
signed on behalf of the Division of Cardiology Professional Standards Committee

c: Physician Peer Review File

Figure 4.2. Example of Physician Letter.

were made only to interventionalists. Although this may appear to be an "easy fix," it required close collaboration and planning with each of the cardiology practices.

An on-call schedule of interventionalists has been developed and posted in the ED, with pictures to assist families in identifying their cardiologist, if applicable. A rotating schedule of interventionalists has been developed for those patients with no preference. Now, when an interventionalist is paged, he/she is given 5 minutes to respond. If he/she does not call back in 5 minutes, he/she is paged again. If there is no response within 5 minutes, the on-call interventionalist is paged. This process has been clearly communicated so that all are aware of it. Individual cases are evaluated on a monthly basis and the process has been refined over time.

Once the team streamlined the hospital's internal processes and removed unnecessary delays in care within in-house, the group began to look at ways to begin the process prior to patient arrival in the ED. The team worked with a large countywide team made up of members of the ambulance companies and area hospitals to develop the capability of obtaining 12-lead electrocardiograms in the field. Completed by emergency medical technicians (EMTs), EKGs can be electronically sent to the ED and available for review by the ED physician. By obtaining EKGs prior to patient arrival, Spectrum Health can determine the presence of a STEMI and activate the STEMI alert process before patient arrival. The interventionalist and the Cath Lab staff can be notified, arrive in the Cath Lab, and be ready to begin the procedure as soon as the patient arrives. This process was designed to be successful no matter what time of day or day of the week.

The ED physician champion was instrumental in working with the emergency medical service (EMS) companies and other hospitals throughout the county to develop a coordinated system for obtaining and transmitting EKGs in the field. Many issues needed to be addressed in this process such as which patients benefit most from this resource, where patients should receive services, what patients should receive fibrinolytics, and how EKGs in the field should be funded.

The latest quality improvement initiative has taken the team outside the health system's boundaries and into the surrounding 13-county region. Spectrum Health has begun to work with local hospitals within the region that do not have a Cath Lab and who refer patients into the Spectrum Heart Center. To streamline the process of transferring STEMI patients quickly for PCI treatment, the team devised a process similar to the in-house process. The group worked with the referring hospitals and ambulance transport companies to develop a STEMI packet and "orange sheet," which standardizes processes and clarifies accountabilities for each member of the team. An integral part of this process was to develop a plan for sharing data and learning between the institutions and ambulance services. To accomplish this, a data agreement needed to be developed between the involved hospitals and ambulance services, a requirement of the Healthcare Information Portability and Accountability Act (HIPAA).

As STEMI patients are identified at outlying hospitals, an "orange sheet" from the STEMI alert packet is initiated. The process is documented as the patient moves from the sending ED, to the ambulance, to Spectrum Health's Cath Lab, to completion of the PCI. The team is developing a process for data analysis and sharing among all involved so that Spectrum can better collaborate for improved patient outcomes. Special attention will be given to determining when it is most beneficial for the patient to receive thrombolytics prior to transport and when it is not.

Although the work of the team is primarily focused on improving care for patients, there is also a financial incentive that plays an important role in focusing the work of the organization and champions. Blue Cross/Blue Shield of Michigan has worked actively with Spectrum Health to set yearly goals and monitor Spectrum Health's attainment of those goals as it relates to time-to-PCI and other core measures. Significant financial reimbursement has been identified and paid out based on achievement of goals. These financial implications have increased the visibility of this work to the Spectrum Health board and are tied to administrator and champion pay-for-performance.

Results

The team's multidisciplinary efforts have led to a significant, sustained decrease in ED arrival-to-PCI times, with a median of 64 minutes and 100% administration of aspirin and beta blockers on arrival. The control charts shown in Figures 4.3 through 4.6 contain some of Spectrum Health's monthly data related to the STEMI project. The observations (shown on the Y axis) are minutes. The numbers in parenthesis (next to the month and year along the X axes of these charts) show how many STEMIs occurred in that month and year. The horizontal lines show upper and lower control limits (UCL and LCL), upper and lower warning limits (UWL and LWL) and the process center line (PCL). Data that fall outside the UWL and LWL are an indicator that the measure is not being met.

Periodic reviews of the data reveal whether Spectrum is achieving its desired level of compliance with the target Joint Commission (and other) measures. If not, the team determines and investigates the cause and an action is taken, such as reporting back to the involved physicians so they can improve their compliance and documentation. These data show that Spectrum is improving the patient care.

Key Elements of Success

Caregivers, by their nature, are eager to work toward goals they perceive as clearly important to improving patient care. They are less willing to strive for improvements they feel do not directly impact patient care and safety. Instrumental to success is sharing the evidence that makes it clear to each member of the team the importance of his/her role in improving outcomes. Members of the ED and Cath Lab, from physician to transport, have a key role that is integral to the patient receiving the best care possible. Sharing the evidence about the importance of rapid time to treatment and outlining each member's role in making that happen, helps team members realize their involvement in improving this process is essential.

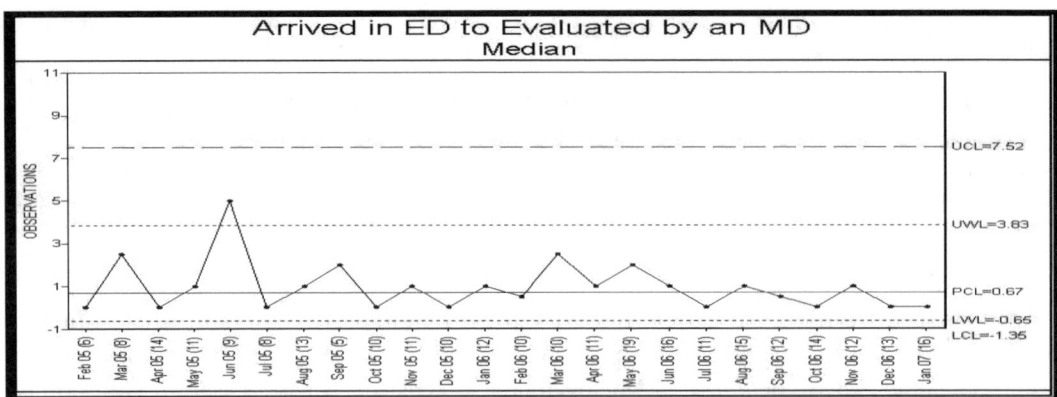

Figure 4.3. Median Time for Arrival in the ED to Be Evaluated by the Physician Has Remained Consistent.

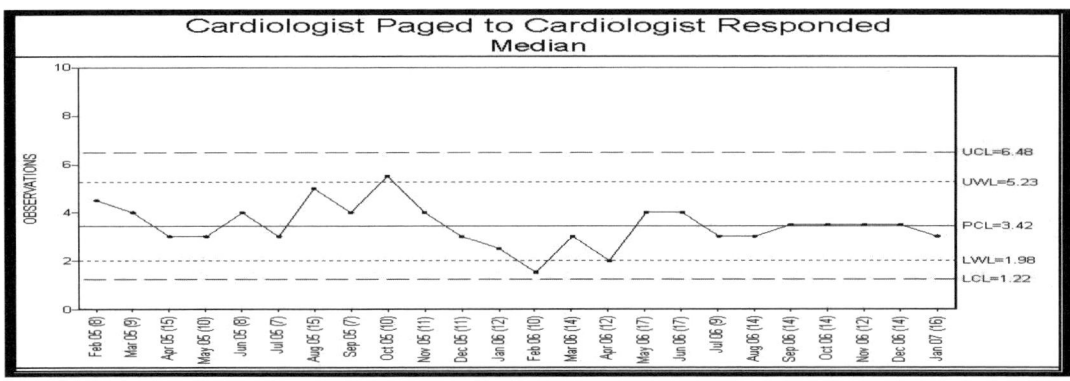

Figure 4.4. The Process for Cardiologist Response Has Become More Stable.

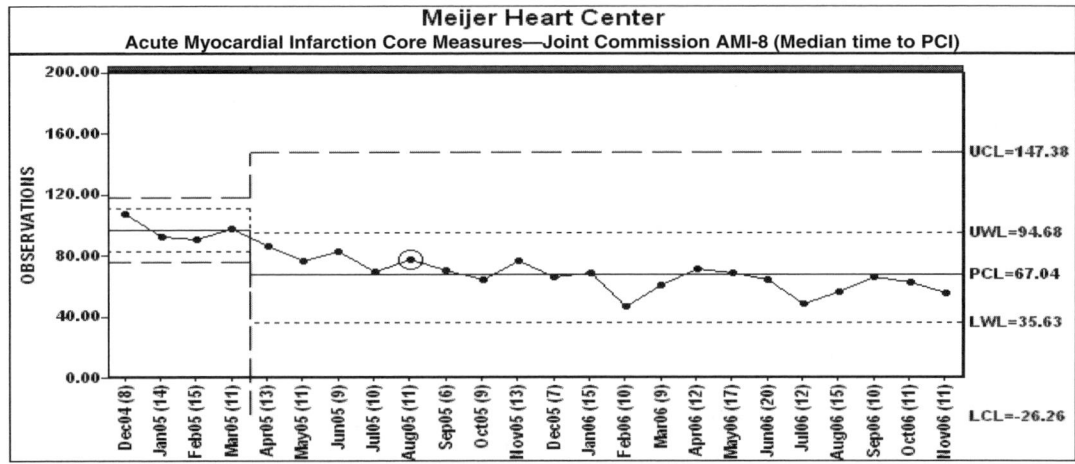

Figure 4.5. The Median Time from Admission in the ED until Balloon Inflation Has Dropped from 98 to 67 Minutes. Real-Time Data Collection through January Shows a Continuing Drop to 61.5 Minutes.

Strong physician and clinical leadership is critical to success. These clinicians must not only champion the concept of reducing door-to-balloon times, but they also must present themselves as the models of cooperation, collaboration, and compromise. One of the elements that helped ensure success of the initiative at Spectrum Health was the extraordinary collaboration among ED and cardiology physicians, and shared team leadership among the emergency, cardiology and quality departments. As the improvement processes continued into the region, that collaborative spirit moved out into the community, with a corresponding need to work closely with other hospitals and EMS.

Strong institutional support for improving processes must be evident from the board of directors, to the administrative team, to the clinical team. A representative from the board was a member of the quality team and data were shared not only with the clinicians, but also in executive forums and board meetings. The data set the tone and expectation that Spectrum was going to achieve its goal and become a regional center of excellence in cardiac care.

Financial incentives were very helpful in focusing efforts on this quality improvement initiative. Although the team remained focused on improving care for patients, Spectrum Health has

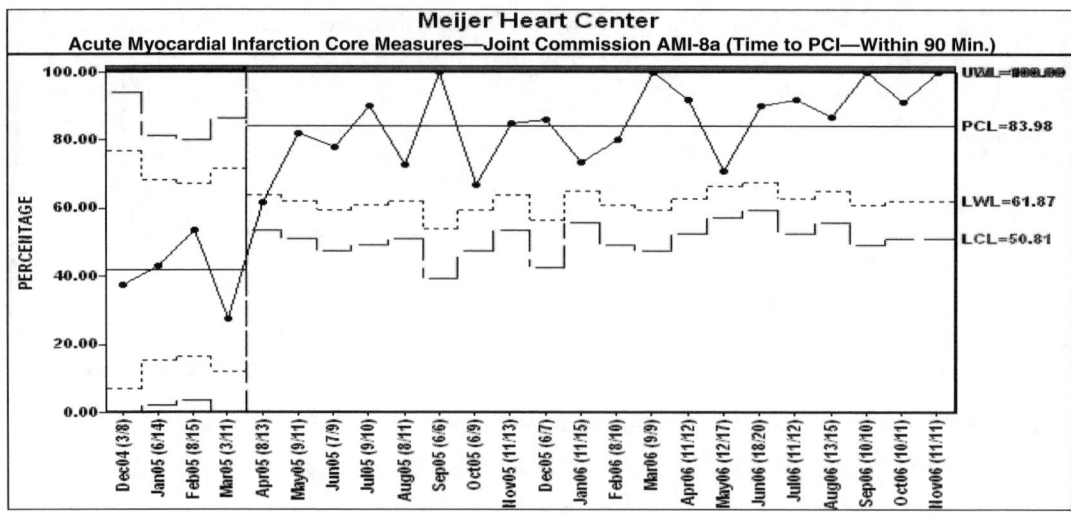

Figure 4.6. Spectrum Continues to Work toward a Goal of Having All STEMI Cases Receive PCI within 90 Minutes of Arrival in the ED. (A significant change in the process occurred in March 2005 with the implementation of the STEMI alert packet.)

been working with Blue Cross/Blue Shield of Michigan to develop a pay-for-performance system based on achieving clearly defined goals. This reimbursement system helps ensure that resources are directed toward success of this effort and maintains a focus on this initiative.

Real-time data collection has helped the team value the data and develop strategies to deal with difficult situations. There is nothing that speaks louder than evidence and data. However, to have real-time data, staff must commit to collecting data consistently and accurately. Missing data elements need to be added and control chart methodology used to help identify and analyze process changes.

The development of standardized processes and clear role delineation was instrumental in helping the team function consistently and dependably. The STEMI alert packet provided the structure necessary to increase efficiency and minimize variation. Accountability for every step of the process should be assigned and the focus of improvement opportunities should be on improving the process, not blaming the practitioner.

Celebrating success should not be an afterthought. It is easy to concentrate on what needs to be changed. It is more difficult to take time out to celebrate what has been accomplished.

Conclusion

The Spectrum Health quality team's improvement process mostly involved taking the components of the larger process apart to find opportunities to incrementally improve the time from door to PCI for these patients. The standardized processes and measurement tools allowed the team to have current data on times and points in the process where improvements needed to be made. The STEMI packet served to "routinize" the processes around treating STEMI patients and made each person in the process aware of what to do and when.

Sharing data with the team increased awareness and fueled the desire to change. In the already nonblaming culture that exists at Spectrum Health, making this data so public and readily available to everyone fostered an air of competition around the process rather than creating fear of punishment for underperformance. The team realized throughout this work what other teams have learned at Spectrum Health: working harder does not necessarily result in process improvements—working smarter is what counts.

References

1. McNamara RL, Herrin J, Bradley EH, et al. NRMI Investigators. Hospital improvement in time to reperfusion in patients with acute myocardial infarction, 1999 to 2002. *J Am Coll Cardiol.* 2006;47:45-51.
2. "What is D2B?" Available at: http://www.d2balliance.org. Accessed January 18, 2007.
3. Bradley EH, Nallamothu BK, Curtis JP, et al. Summary of evidence regarding hospital strategies to reduce door-to-balloon times for patients with ST-segment elevation myocardial infarction undergoing primary percutaneous coronary intervention. *Crit Pathw Cardiol.* 2007;6:91-97.

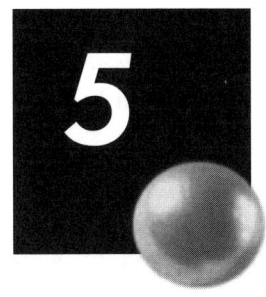

Clostridium difficile–Associated Disease: Time to Press the Panic Button?

Pazit Shaked

The Hospital

St. Mary Medical Center (SMMC) is a 327-bed, nonteaching level II trauma, community hospital located on the outskirts of Philadelphia. The hospital serves mostly the adult population. Besides internal medicine, labor and delivery, and general surgery, the hospital focuses heavily on cardiac services. Other growing service lines include orthopedic surgery. The hospital has a busy same-day-surgery operation. Transplant surgery is not available.

Background

The incidence and severity of *Clostridium difficile*–associated diarrhea has been increasing throughout the United States. These new cases are more severe cases associated with an increase in mortality. The Centers for Disease Control and Prevention (CDC) has reported cases in previously healthy individuals once thought to be at low risk for this disease, such as children and postpartum women.[1]

U.S. hospital discharges for which *Clostridium difficile*–associated disease (CDAD) was listed as any diagnosis nearly doubled from 82,000 (95% confidence interval [CI] 71,000–94,000) or 31/100,000 population in 1996 to 178,000 (95% CI 151,000–205,000) or 61/100,000 in 2003; this increase was significant between 2000 and 2003 (slope of linear trend 9.48; 95% CI 6.16–12.80, $p = 0.01$).[2] The overall infection rate during this period was much higher in people 65 years of age or older (228/100,000) than in the age group with the next highest rate, 45–64 years (40/100,000; $p<0.001$).[2] Between 1987–1998 CDC data show there were 12.2 cases per 10,000 patient days.[3]

Antibiotic therapy represents a significant risk factor for development of CDAD.[3] Further, the risk of developing this disease increases with multiple antibiotics and longer treatment duration.[4] Recently, the number and severity of CDAD cases has increased at SMMC. Many of these patients required surgical intervention. Moreover, there have been deaths at SMMC linked to *C. difficile* diarrhea. Pharmacy leadership at SMMC decided to undertake a clinical intervention to reduce the incidence of *C. difficile* diarrhea. SMMC data before initiation of this project showed 25 to 32 cases of hospital-acquired CDAD per 10,000 patient days.

The Intervention

According to the CDC, one of the key interventions necessary to control the spread of *C. difficile* is judicious use of antibiotics. Clinical pharmacy activities and involvement at SMMC indicated that there was an opportunity to decrease the use of broad spectrum antibiotics as well as decrease the duration of antibiotic therapy. The initial plan developed by the pharmacy department included two proposals:

1. **1-day expiration on postoperative antibiotics** (excluding orders for patients who had undergone drainage of an abscess, had a ruptured colon, had an emergent cholecystectomy with suspected peritonitis, or had sinus surgery). Pharmacy personnel would review these orders for appropriateness, taking corrective action as needed.

2. **5-day expiration on all antibiotics prescribed by non-infectious disease (ID) physicians.** Antibiotic renewals would be screened retrospectively, using the pharmacy computer system, for legitimacy.

As the first phase of the intervention (June 2006), the pharmacy began the automatic stop of postoperative antibiotics. Specifically, the program was implemented by pharmacy students during weekdays and supervised by the pharmacy clinical coordinator. Recommendations were based on published guidelines from the American Society of Health System-Pharmacists (ASHP), Infectious Disease Society of America (IDSA), and CDC regarding the proper utilization of antimicrobials as surgical prophylaxis.

Unfortunately, every good thing has an end. Although this program was approved by SMMC's Medical Executive Committee, it had to be stopped within the first month due to physician objection. The second part of the program as outlined above was not implemented. Despite the difficulty that arose, the pharmacy department revised the intervention so pharmacy students assigned to SMMC on an ID rotation left written communications for physicians as follows:

- Recommendations to discontinue antibiotics (either due to a lack of indication or completed course)
- Recommendations to narrow antibiotics spectrum based on culture results

During the first few days of each infectious disease rotation, students learned the surveillance system. The pharmacy department created reports of all patients receiving antimicrobials (oral and injectables). The students used standardized data collection forms to record patients' antimicrobial history (including preadmission treatment), the indication for therapy according to the prescriber, any data that could be used to support this diagnosis (such as vital signs, hematology lab data, or microbiology lab data) and the plan for therapy as indicated in the physician progress notes. The student then made his/her own assessment regarding the appropriateness of the antibiotic therapy. Any cases where interventions were warranted were reviewed by the preceptor, and the action plan was discussed. Students were empowered to make independent decisions regarding route change (from IV to PO).

Challenges

Several issues arose with the pharmacy's ability to implement even this modified program completely. First was the lack of continuity among ID pharmacy students rotating through SMMC. ID students were not sent to SMMC every month, so there were some months when the program was not able to be executed. The second issue was the learning curve each pharmacy student faced at the beginning of each 5-week ID rotation. The students had to understand the surveillance system, be proficient and efficient at using the pharmacy computer system and collecting the applicable data from the paper charts and the computer and, most importantly, review and be familiar with any infectious diseases and surgery types that were involved in their cases in order to be able to exert critical judgment and make clinical recommendations. Both factors affected the efficiency of the surveillance program. Also, pharmacy students who rotated to SMMC earlier in the year did not have the same degree of clinical skill and experience as their counterparts who rotated into the service later in the year, further compromising program consistency.

Results

The change in CDAD at the hospital is shown in Figure 5.1. Over time, there has been a trend of decreased rates of nosocomial *C. difficile* infections. However, due to the issues previously discussed, the success of the program has fluctuated with the ability of the pharmacy students to perform the surveillance.

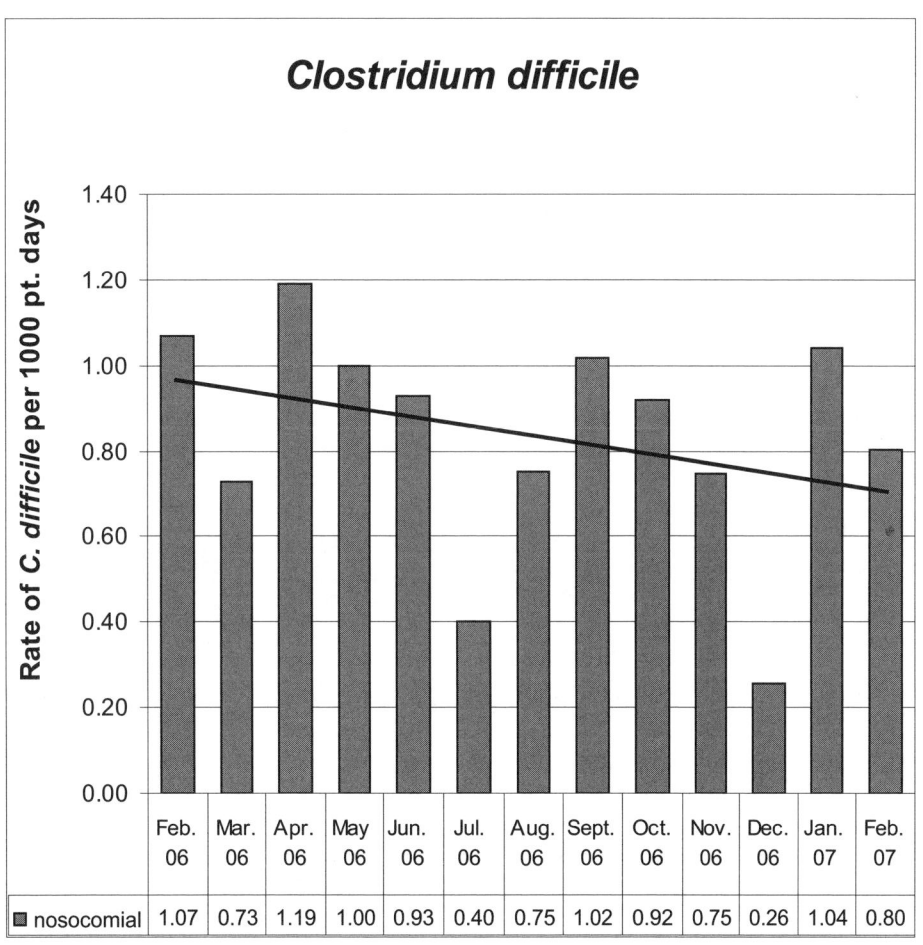

	Feb. 06	Mar. 06	Apr. 06	May 06	Jun. 06	Jul. 06	Aug. 06	Sept. 06	Oct. 06	Nov. 06	Dec. 06	Jan. 07	Feb. 07
■ nosocomial	1.07	0.73	1.19	1.00	0.93	0.40	0.75	1.02	0.92	0.75	0.26	1.04	0.80

Figure 5.1. SMMC Monthly *C. difficile* Infection Rate.

Conclusion

The current observational project raises the possibility that a systematic intervention for judicious use of antibiotics in the hospital setting may decrease the rates of nosocomial *C. difficile*–associated disease. Randomized controlled studies are needed in order to assess the true merit of such an intervention.

References

1. Centers for Disease Control and Prevention. Chernak E, Johnson CC, Weltman A, et al. Severe Clostridium difficile—associated disease in populations previously at low risk—four states, 2005. *MMWR*. 2005;54:1201-1205. Available at: http://www.cdc.gov/mmwr/preview/ mmwrhtml/mm5447a1.htm. Accessed September 2007.
2. McDonald LC, Owings M, Jernigan DB. Clostridium difficile infection in patients discharged from U.S. short-stay hospitals, 1996–2003. *Emerg Infect Dis*. [serial on the Internet]. Available at: http://www.cdc.gov/ncidod/EID/vol12no03/05-1064.htm. Accessed September 2007.
3. Sunenshine RH, McDonald LC. Clostridium difficile associated diarrhea: new challenges from an established pathogen. *CCJM*. 2006;73:187-197.
4. Pepin J, Saheb N, Coulombe MA, et al. Emergence of fluoroquinolones as the predominant risk factor for Clostridium difficile–associated diarrhea: a cohort study during an epidemic in Quebec. *Clin Infect Dis*. 2005;41:1254-1260.

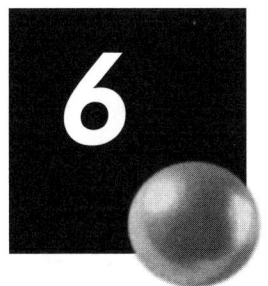

Pneumonia Core Measures: Tools Used by Pharmacy to Help Ensure Adherence

Kelly C. A. Ervin
Susan J. Skledar

The Setting

The University of Pittsburgh Medical Center (UPMC) is an academic, multifacility healthcare system. Comprised of 19 hospitals with multiple care sites across western Pennsylvania and throughout the world, UPMC also offers a growing health insurance product.

The UPMC Presbyterian Shadyside is a medical-surgical facility located in Pittsburgh, Pennsylvania and is situated on the Oakland Campus of the University of Pittsburgh, Schools of Health Sciences. UPMC Presbyterian is a leading center for organ transplantation, cardiology, cardiothoracic surgery, critical care medicine, geriatrics, neurosurgery, oncology, primary care, psychiatry, and trauma services. The pharmacy department at UPMC Presbyterian offers a variety of services, including clinical pharmacist/faculty coverage to the above-mentioned areas, anesthesiology/operating room satellite pharmacies, automated dispensing systems, a decentralized pharmacy care model, an investigational drug service , a unit-dose intravenous admixture program that is fully computerized, and a Drug Use and Disease State Management (DUDSM) program that is nationally recognized.[1] The UPMC Presbyterian DUDSM Program was developed to evaluate opportunities for optimizing pharmacotherapy and design evidence-based drug use and disease state management algorithms and clinical practice guidelines.[1]

Pneumonia and Core Measure Quality Indicators

In the United States, community-acquired pneumonia (CAP), along with influenza, is the seventh leading cause of death.[2,3] Mortality rates have not significantly declined for these diseases despite many efforts, including increased national focus, preventative health programs, advances in antibiotic therapy, changes in care processes, and availability of national guidelines.[2]

With the national focus from the Centers for Medicare and Medicaid Services (CMS) and the Joint Commission™, as well as a regional focus in Pennsylvania, UPMC set an internal target of 90% compliance with the following pneumonia core measure indicators[4,5]:

- Blood cultures, if drawn, should be done prior to initiating antibiotic therapy.
- Assessment of oxygenation by arterial blood gas monitoring or pulse oximetry should be done within 8 hours after admission.
- Antibiotic therapy should be initiated within 4 hours of hospital arrival.
- Initial antibiotic selection must be in accordance with published guidelines.

- Smoking cessation information should be provided to patients who smoke.

- Pneumococcal polysaccharide and influenza vaccine should be administered before discharge.

As with all hospitals, core measure indicators are reported in a public domain at http://www.hospitalcompare.hhs.gov.

Tasked with improving care of patients with pneumonia (particularly CAP), DUDSM staff and other healthcare professionals at the hospital formed an interdisciplinary CAP workgroup. The workgroup functioned to create and implement processes for monitoring and ensuring compliance with the pneumonia core measures established by the CMS and the Joint Commission.[4,5] At UPMC Presbyterian, it was also necessary to ensure compliance with the Pennsylvania Elderly Immunization Act, which requires hospitals to offer immunizations to elderly inpatients prior to their discharge.[6]

Compliance Monitoring

A variety of monitoring processes were implemented to meet the core measure indicators. For example, informatics tools, such as the reports shown in Table 6.1, were designed to help identify CAP patients on a daily basis. The reports included a pneumonia/respiratory admission diagnosis code report, generated from the UPMC medical archive database. Also, pharmacy personnel created a drug utilization report listing antimicrobials likely to be used in the treatment of CAP (e.g., azithromycin, ceftriaxone, moxifloxacin) and a daily new admission list sorted by age to identify patients greater than or equal to 65 years old. The drug utilization report was created to capture patients who may not have been identified in the diagnosis code report—those that developed pneumonia later in their admission process, for example. There was also a daily patient transfer report that identified patients with orders for influenza or pneumococcal polysaccharide vaccines that had not been administered before being transferred to another unit.

These reports are reviewed daily in the pharmacy. Pharmacists are permitted by hospital policy to order vaccines on eligible patients, following patient-specific risk assessment criteria (which includes an evaluation of prior vaccine administration). The data analyst pharmacy technician and student pharmacists perform the daily review of the reports and prepare the initial orders for pharmacist

Table 6.1. Daily Computer Reports and Their Functions

Report	Function
Pneumonia admission DRG	Identifies new patients with diagnoses related to CAP, regardless of age
Antibiotic drug use evaluation	Identifies patients that were ordered CAP-related antibiotics after admission, signifying a possible CAP diagnosis
Admissions from the last 24 hr	Identifies all patients that were admitted within the last 24 hr sorted by date of birth; used for identification of the elderly
Transferred patients to and from intensive care units	Identifies patients with orders for vaccines that were not administered prior to transfer; allows pharmacists to rewrite orders

evaluation. The complete process for the UPMC inpatient standing orders program for vaccination has been described elsewhere.[7,8]

To improve compliance with the indicator measure related to timeliness of antibiotic administration, the emergency department (ED) admission process was expanded to include all hospital admissions with pneumonia, including those admitted directly from outpatient physician offices. This policy change facilitated first-antibiotic-dose administration in the ED. Regarding vaccine administration, the pharmacy generates daily reports for nursing directors of inpatient units. These reports identify which patients should receive an influenza and/or pneumonia polysaccharide vaccine on the given day. Use of these reports help ensure vaccine administration and appropriate documentation, such as whether the vaccine was actually given, refused by the patient, or not needed because the patient reported having already received the vaccination in the outpatient setting.

Pharmacy students or pharmacy technicians document current or prior vaccine administration in the immunization portion of the electronic health record. Nurses are required to document vaccine lot number, expiration date, site and date of administration in electronic medication administration record. To stimulate more consistent documentation of UPMC patients' vaccination status on admission, the inpatient nursing admission/history intake forms were updated to include a reminder to ask patients about their immunizations. This information is easily accessed by the pharmacy during the patient screening process.

The multidisciplinary work group meets monthly to improve care standards and focus on variances from core measure targets. Physician champions from the work group consistently educate the medical staff about the pneumonia core measures and what UPMC is doing to achieve compliance with them. Further, a clinical nurse specialist rounds daily on core measures patients to ensure processes are complete on all patients. This nurse and the pharmacy staff provide real-time education to bedside nurses regarding the care of CAP patients and related UPMC processes.

Implementation Tools

There are a variety of tools that have facilitated efforts to achieve the targeted core measure compliance. An established evidence-based hospital guideline for management of the patient of CAP has been implemented, derived from the latest published guidelines.[2] The guideline recommends empiric antimicrobial therapy with azithromycin plus ceftriaxone, and also indicates that patients should be vaccinated prior to hospital discharge. The workgroup physician champion conducts focused education about this core measure to the ED and internal medicine healthcare team. This education reinforces the evidence and importance of appropriate management of the patient with CAP. A hospital preprinted order form for CAP has also been implemented to help guide care of these patients.

From a process perspective, first doses of antibiotics likely to be used in the treatment of CAP (mentioned above) are stored and obtained by the nurse, under direction of the ED physician, from the ED automated medication cabinets. Placing these antibiotic doses in the ED has helped both with appropriate antimicrobial selection and first-dose timing.

To ensure consistent screening processes and documentation in the medical record, the pharmacists use a vaccine order form to initiate pneumococcal polysaccharide vaccine (see Figure 6.1); a similar form is available for influenza vaccine. Since UPMC nurses provide smoking cessation materials to all admitted patients, nursing leadership designed a Healthy Lifestyle Brochure (see Figure 6.2) to educate all patients against the dangers of smoking and to offer smoking cessation advice.

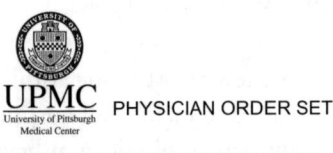

PHYSICIAN ORDER SET

University of Pittsburgh
Medical Center

AUTHORIZATION IS GIVEN TO THE PHARMACY TO DISPENSE AND TO THE

NURSE TO ADMINISTER THE GENERIC OR CHEMICAL EQUIVALENT WHEN

THE DRUG IS FILLED BY THE PHARMACY OF THE UPMC HEALTH SYSTEM

HOSPITAL–UNLESS THE PRODUCT NAME IS CIRCLED.

IMPRINT PATIENT IDENTIFICATION HERE

Pneumococcal Polysaccharide Vaccine Assessment and Standing Order Form

Check all boxes that apply with a ☒

Risk Assessment–No Active Orders	Order Section
Step 1: Determine the patient's risk:	☐ Administer pneumococcal polysaccharide vaccine 0.5 mL:
☐ Age: 65 years. **Proceed to Step 2.**	☐ deep IM in deltoid
☐ Age 2–64 years with any of the following:	☐ Subcutaneous if INR >1.5 or platelets <100,000
Chronic Illnesses: cardiovascular disease, pulmonary disease	☐ Subcutaneous if patient is on heparin drip or warfarin
(not asthma), diabetes mellitus, alcoholism, liver disease,	
sickle cell anemia, cerebrospinal fluid leaks, cochlear implant	and give:
recipients, **and/or**	☐ Now
is *immunocompromised*: HIV infection, leukemia, lymphoma,	☐ on at _____ :00
Hodgkins disease, multiple myeloma, generalized malignancy,	
asplenic, chronic renal failure, nephrotic syndrome, organ or	
bone marrow transplantation, immunosuppressive medications	☐ Do NOT administer pneumococcal vaccine.
Proceed to Step 2	
☐ Age 2–64 years and an Alaskan native or of other Native	
American descent. **Proceed to Step 2.**	
☐ Age 2–64 years with no risk factors. **Proceed to Order Section**	
and check "do not administer vaccine" box.	
Step 2: Assess for contraindications:	
☐ Hypersensitivity to vaccine component.	
Proceed to Order Section and check "do not administer	
vaccine" box	
☐ Severe reaction to prior pneumococcal vaccine.	
Proceed to Order Section and check "do not administer	
vaccine" box	
☐ Patient received chemotherapy within the last three months or may	
receive chemotherapy within two weeks.	
Proceed to Order Section and check "do not administer	
vaccine" box	Signature: _____
☐ Patient's vaccinations are evaluated and administered in	
outpatient clinic/office	
Proceed to Order Section and check "do not administer	Printed Name: _____
vaccine" box	
☐ No contraindications noted from available information:	
Proceed to Step 3.	Pager/phone: _____
Step 3: Assess previous vaccination history:	
☐ Uncertain or unknown status. **Proceed to Order Section**	Date: _____
and check "administer vaccine" box	

IPO   Form ID: PUH/SHY-1383 Last Revision Date: 9/10/2007

Figure 6.1. Pneumococcal Polysaccharide Vaccine Assessment and Standing Order Form.

Results

As of the current fiscal year, UPMC has met or exceeded the >90% compliance goal for the pneumonia core measures and the vaccine program immunization rates in the elderly (see Table 6.2).

ingredients. Many cause cancers.

☹ Cigarette smoking/secondhand smoke cause: shortness of breath, decreased energy, bone loss, damaged blood vessels, lung cancer, other cancers, high blood pressure, digestive disorders, diabetes complications, chronic lung diseases, heart disease, impaired circulation ...

☹ Cigarette smoking ruins clothing, furniture, car seats, as well as family and social relationships

☹ Cost of cigarettes averages $4/pack

☹ Medical costs of smoking related diseases = over $50 billion annually

☹ Lost wages and productivity: another $50 billion annually

☹ Parental smoking causes low birth weight, premature deaths and increases risk of Sudden Infant Death Syndrome among newborns and increases risk of learning disabilities

☹ Asthma, Bronchitis, respiratory and ear infections increase in children of smokers

☹ Parental smoking causes 6,200 children deaths per year from infections and burns

☹ Cigarette smoking: a major cause of fire deaths

☹ Matches and lighters: Major causes of house fires

> **Over 5,000 children per day try smoking, 3,000 become *hooked***

End the Bad News ...

"Preventing Smoking among young people is critical to ending the **EPIDEMIC** of tobacco use ... "

—Centers for Disease Control

Good News ... Quitting

☺ Immediately after your last cigarette:

- No more burns in clothes, furniture, car, fingers ...
- Healing processes begin

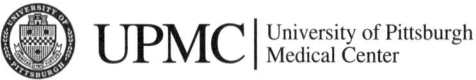

UPMC | University of Pittsburgh Medical Center

Healthy Lifestyle

We at UPMC are committed to providing you with the highest quality of care. While you are hospitalized, a number of health care team members will meet with you to provide you with teaching about your condition and health.

This brochure contains some general recommendations and guidelines for your continued health and well being.

If you have questions about your hospitalization while here or after you are discharged, our Patient and Family Support Services is available to assist you. A patient relations representative is available at [phone number]. *Please contact us at anytime with questions or concerns.*

Figure 6.2. Excerpt from Healthy Lifestyle Brochure.

Table 6.2. Yearly Pneumonia Core Measures Compliance Rates

	FY04	FY05	FY06	FY07
Assessment of oxygenation within 24 hr after admission	98.3	99.8	99.5	100
Blood cultures (if drawn) should be drawn prior to initiating antibiotic therapy	73.7	82.8	94.8	96.2
Antibiotic therapy should be initiated within 4 hr of hospital arrival	Data not reported	73.7	75.4	92.8
Antibiotic selection according to guidelines	Data not reported	56.9%	81.3	93.1
Smoking cessation information should be provided to patients who smoke	42	78.6	97.2	94.5
Pneumococcal polysaccharide vaccine provided to patient before discharge[a]	21.5	75	89.1	90.4

[a]Influenza vaccination rate for FY06 = 72.6% and FY07 = 76.6%.

Conclusions

Since achievement of pneumonia core measures is mandated by CMS and the Joint Commission, processes and tools have been implemented to help ensure compliance with these quality measures. Daily monitoring and intervention by a designated team of healthcare professionals ensured compliance with guidelines at UPMC Presbyterian and allowed for real-time education at the point of care. Although this effort requires dedicated resources, it has allowed top-tier reporting for all core measures. Continued actions involve better front-line staff awareness of this program and automatic screening processes for core measure patient identification with physician order-entry technology.

References

1. Skledar SJ, Hess MM. Implementation of a drug-use and disease state management program. *Am J Health Syst Pharm.* 2000;57(suppl 4):S23-S29.

2. Mandell LA, Wunderink RG, Anzueto A, et al. Infectious Diseases Society of America/American Thoracic Society Consensus Guidelines on the Management of Community-Acquired Pneumonia in Adults. *Clin Infect Dis.* 2007;44:S27-S72.

3. National Center for Health Statistics. Health, United States, 2006, with chartbook on trends in the health of Americans. Available at: http://www.cdc.gov/nchs/data/hus/hus06.pdf. Accessed September 20, 2007.

4. Performance Measurement Initiatives. The Joint Commission. Available at: http://www.jointcommission.org/PerformanceMeasurement/PerformanceMeasurement/Pneumonia+Core+Measure+Set.htm. Accessed September 20, 2007.

5. Pneumonia. MedQIC. Available at: http://medqic.org/dcs/ContentServer?cid=1089815967023&pagename=Medqic%2FContent%2FParentShellTemplate&parentName=Topic&c=MQParents. Accessed September 20, 2007.

6. The Pennsylvania Department of Health. The elderly immunization act: Act 86. Available at: www.dsf.health.state.pa.us/health/lib/health/flu/senate_bill_769.pdf. Accessed January 20, 2005.

7. Sokos DR, Skledar SJ, Ervin KA, et al. Designing and implementing a hospital-based vaccine standing orders program. *Am J Health Syst Pharm.* 2007;64:1096-1102.

8. Skledar SJ, McKaveney TP, Sokos DR, et al. Role of student pharmacist interns in hospital-based standing orders pneumococcal vaccination program. *J Am Pharm Assoc.* 2007;47:404-409.

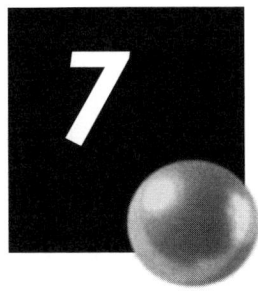

2-4-6-8, Sliding Scale's Not Really Great!

Rebecca Garner

Heather Myers Huentelman

Acknowledgments: The authors would like to recognize the additional members of the interdisciplinary team that implemented the performance improvement project to improve glycemic control in the inpatient setting including Daniel Diggins, Pharm.D., Marie Russell, MD, Gerald Bush, MD, and Jeremy Graham, MD.

Learning Objective

The learning objective is to review the benefits of basal insulin versus "sliding scale" insulin in the treatment of inpatients with diabetes.

About the Facility

Phoenix Indian Medical Center (PIMC) is an urban, 110-bed, government hospital based in Phoenix, Arizona. On the inpatient wards there are approximately 4,700 admissions per year. This facility serves a primarily Native American population from the local Phoenix area and is also the main referral center for many outlying Indian Health Service facilities in Arizona, Nevada, Utah, and California.*

The inpatient pharmacy staff at PIMC consists of six full-time clinical pharmacists; two full-time "floater" pharmacists trained for inpatient and outpatient work; and one postgraduate year one (PGY-1) pharmacy resident, who spends about 5 months per year on inpatient assignments and the rest of the time on outpatient services. In 2004, the pharmacy resident determined that there was room for improvement in the way the medical center controlled the blood glucoses of its diabetic wound patients. Developing and implementing a successful protocol for providing intensive glycemic control for this subset of patients became her mission in life (at least it felt that way to her)!

How Long Does Insulin's Effect Last?

Let's take a step back in time (for most of us) and review some basic things taught in pharmacy school about insulin. Exogenous insulin is administered in an attempt to mimic the body's normal secretion of insulin or overcome insulin resistance. Basal insulin administration is meant to replace the insulin that is lacking from either missing or declining beta-cell function of the pancreas, in a

---

Disclaimer: The views expressed do not necessarily represent the views of the Public Health Service or the United States.

*Data obtained from PIMC's Resource and Patient Management System, August 2007.

manner that provides a more constant level of insulin. This replacement can be achieved by supplying intermediate- or long-acting insulin formulations given intermittently, or short-acting insulin given as a continuous infusion.[1] Insulins can be broadly categorized by the length of time that they are active in the body and able to have blood glucose lowering effects.

As seen in Figure 7.1, rapid-acting insulins, such as those used for sliding scale administration, would produce a "see-saw" effect if dosed intermittently as monotherapy throughout the day.

What Is Sliding Scale Insulin (SSI)?

The term *sliding scale insulin* refers to the use of a variable dose of short-acting insulin, given intermittently at intervals determined by a prescriber in response to an individual blood glucose measurement (usually by fingerstick method). Most commonly, fingerstick glucose measurements are taken "every 6 hours" or "30 minutes before meals and bedtime." A common formula for calculating the short-acting insulin sliding scale dose is

Number of units insulin = (blood glucose – 200) divided by 10 (or 20)

Testing this formula with some possible glucose values will demonstrate that this formula does not even begin to correct for elevated glucose levels until they reach 210 mg/dL [e.g., (glucose 210–200)/10 = 1 unit regular insulin]. (Normal blood glucose levels range from 70–110 mg/dL.) The nurses at PIMC are unlikely to actually administer 1 unit of insulin (equal to 0.1 mL of U-100 insulin). Usually, PIMC's nurses will not administer the sliding scale insulin until the patient's blood glucose reading is high enough to make the dose a reasonably measurable amount.

Some sliding scale regimens initiate treatment earlier at lower glucose values than the standard formulas and are more patient-specific. Table 7.1 provides an example. Alternatively, there are also weight-based nomograms for determining SSI doses.[2] Although all of these methods share some major drawbacks, they definitely decrease the numbers of phone calls to prescribers about elevated glucose values.

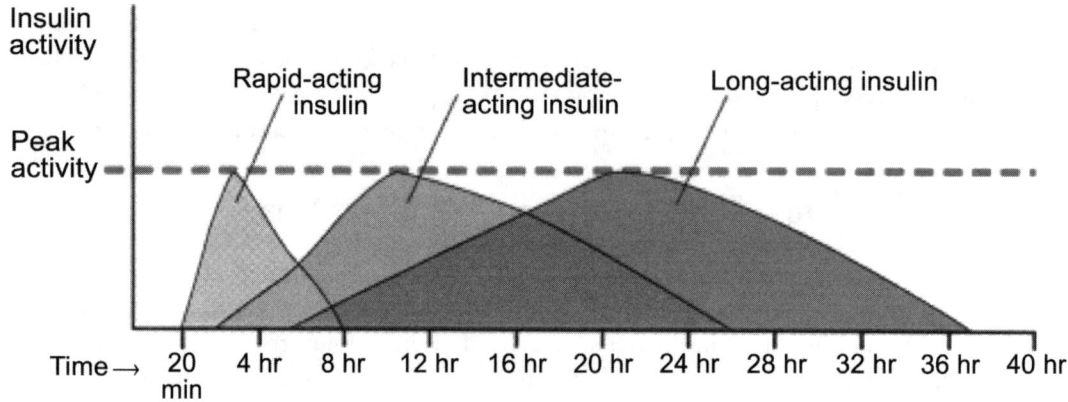

Figure 7.1. Characteristics of Insulins.
Source: Beers MH, ed. *The Merck Manual of Medical Information, Second Home Edition.* Whitehouse Station, NJ: Merck & Co Inc; 2003:967. Available at: www.merck.com/mmhe/sec13/ch165/ch165a.html. Accessed August 15, 2007. Permission obtained for use.

Table 7.1. Sliding Scale Insulin Dose (given subcutaneously)

Glucose 0–80, call provider
Glucose 80–150, give 0 units
Glucose 151–200, give 2 units
Glucose 201–250, give 4 units
Glucose 251–300, give 6 units
Glucose 301–350, give 8 units
If glucose over 350, give 10 units and call provider

What's Wrong with Using Sliding Scale Insulin?

The American Association of Clinical Endocrinologists published a Position Statement on the benefits of providing intensive glycemic control for inpatients,

> "Effective insulin therapy must provide both basal and nutritional meal and/or intravenous glucose coverage in order to achieve the target goals. Hospitalized patients often require high insulin doses to achieve desired target glucose levels. In addition to basal and nutritional insulin requirements, patients often require supplemental or correction insulin for treatment of unexpected hyperglycemia. Use of "sliding scale" insulin alone is discouraged; evidence does not support this technique because it has resulted in unacceptably high rates of hyperglycemia, hypoglycemia, and iatrogenic diabetic ketoacidosis in hospitalized patients. The use of standardized protocols that are developed by multidisciplinary teams is associated with improved glycemic control and lower rates of hypoglycemia. In addition to specifying insulin dose, protocols should also include specific guidelines for identifying patients at risk for hypoglycemia and actions to be taken to prevent and treat hypoglycemia."[3]

Besides allowing blood glucose levels to become unacceptably elevated (e.g., 210 mg/dL) before correction, SSI does not take into account the relationship of blood glucose to dietary intake. If a patient is not eating (NPO) or is receiving tube feedings, the times and amounts of nutrition can vary widely. An isolated high glucose value could be inappropriately treated with the use of SSI while a patient is NPO and not on appropriate monitoring or intravenous fluids. It is easy to make a patient NPO for a procedure, then forget to address the existing SSI or scheduled insulin orders.

Times for fingerstick glucose measurements vary between facilities, since meal times vary. Often patients are fed three times daily and not given food after the (5 p.m.) evening meal unless they request a snack. In this scenario, if (short-acting) SSI is given at the evening meal and again at bedtime for elevated glucose levels but no caloric intake is given, the possibility of nighttime hypoglycemia is very real, as is the chance of morning hyperglycemia once the short-acting insulin wears off. Another pitfall is if a glucose measurement is taken and a dose of SSI is given 30 minutes before the planned mealtime, and then the meal tray does not come, is delayed, or the patient does not want to eat; the insulin will continue to work, potentially resulting in hypoglycemia.

Finally, the use of SSI is reactive rather than proactive, meaning that one must wait until the blood glucose is high to begin to take action to lower the glucose. Several studies have demonstrated increased hyperglycemic episodes with sliding scale insulin regimens, and that there are potential negative consequences for using solely intermittent short-acting insulin.[4]

Project Goal

The goal of the project was to decrease patients' daily fluctuations and high blood glucose values by providing adequate basal insulin levels through implementation of a standardized, safe, and effective protocol for subcutaneous insulin management. The study team believed regulation of patients' blood glucose levels would improve wound healing, decrease infections, minimize length of stay, and decrease overall healthcare costs.[5,6] The protocol included inpatient medicine and surgery service patients, to see what improvements in blood glucose control could be achieved.

Reason for Intervention

American Indians and Alaska Natives continue to be disproportionately diagnosed with diabetes. Current data published in June 2007 put rates of diabetes diagnosis at 16.3% for American Indians and Alaska Natives compared with 8.7% of non-Hispanic whites.[7] Diabetes as a comorbidity occurs nationally in 10% to 30% of hospitalized patients. However, at PIMC the rate is much higher; 35% of hospitalized patients were diabetics in 2000 and an estimated 45% of hospitalized patients were diabetics in 2004. With the high incidence of diabetes in the Native population, this specific performance improvement project was undertaken after the release of the American College of Endocrinology Task Force position statement on inpatient diabetes and metabolic control.[3] The position statement was based on current literature that demonstrated controlling hyperglycemia in acute care patients with insulin infusion decreased morbidity, mortality, and length of stay. These benefits were seen regardless of whether the person had been previously diagnosed with diabetes.

PIMC decided to assess the current diabetes control of its hospitalized patients and to determine if the control could be improved through a reproducible protocol. In September 2004, 40% of hospitalized diabetic patients in the medical and surgical units (nonintensive care units) had average blood glucose levels greater than 160 mg/dL. It was determined that glycemic control could be improved. However, due to staffing and monitoring issues, the use of insulin infusion was not available to patients outside the intensive care unit. This lack of continuously infused insulin limited the intervention to subcutaneous insulin.

Literature has shown that protocols improve diabetes care over physician intuition.[8,9] The Joint Commission™ supports using standardized protocols for glycemic control rather than individualized sliding scales. This project specifically meets Joint Commission National Patient Safety Goal 3 (improving the safety of using medication in the hospital setting).[10] The protocol was developed to standardize care and potentially decrease overall healthcare costs (i.e., through the decreased incidence of certain diabetic complications) while improving patient outcomes. The pervasive thought that it is acceptable to let patients "run a little sweet," can actually cause harm to patients by increasing infection rates, wound healing time, and lengths of stay. Accordingly, managing hyperglycemia was determined to be a priority for all hospitalized patients and a standardized subcutaneous insulin protocol was designed and implemented.

Protocol Description

A subcutaneous insulin protocol was developed by an interdisciplinary team of internal medicine physicians and clinical pharmacists based on published literature and protocols from local hospitals. The protocol was reviewed by hospital staff including physicians, nurses, diabetes educators, and pharmacists. The targeted population was adult noncritical medicine/surgery patients with two blood glucose readings over 200 mg/dL in 24 hours. The comparison group was adult noncritical medicine/surgery patients treated with any combination of oral diabetic medications and insulin (standard care).

Insulin Adjustments

Patients with two or more blood glucose readings greater than 200 mg/dL in a 24-hour period were identified by consultation or review of inpatient electronic records. These patients were started on the subcutaneous insulin protocol. The members of the team met daily to review all patients being managed by the protocol and to make dosing adjustments. Blood glucose goals were 80–120 mg/dL (fasting) and 90–160 mg/dL (random). Starting insulin doses were calculated based on home insulin dose, inpatient insulin use (sliding scale or infusion), or body mass index (BMI). This total daily insulin (TDI) was initially administered as basal insulin (glargine insulin 40% of TDI) and prandial insulin (regular insulin 60% of TDI, divided three times daily 30 minutes prior to meals). Additional supplemental insulin was given for hyperglycemia and added to prandial insulin requirements. TDI was decreased by 10% to 20% for blood glucose levels less than 80 mg/dL and increased by 10% to 20% for blood glucose levels greater than 180 mg/dL. Blood glucose was monitored prior to meals, bedtime, and if patients had suspected or symptomatic hypoglycemia. Glargine was decreased by 10% for NPO status and prandial regular insulin was held.

The implementation and management of the protocol was conducted by an interdisciplinary diabetes management team. This performance improvement project was implemented in January 2005, and results were evaluated in April of 2005. The primary goal was to determine if the standardized subcutaneous insulin protocol improved glycemic control over standard care.

Evaluation

Data collected included incidence of hypoglycemia and hyperglycemia, type of insulin used, and time within the goal blood glucose range. Adherence to baseline evaluations recommended by inpatient diabetes management guidelines, such as lipid profiles, glycosylated hemoglobin (HbA1C), urinary analysis, microalbumin, and electrocardiogram were also recorded.[11] This information was used to determine the overall effectiveness and safety of the proposed protocol. Since literature has demonstrated improved outcomes with better glycemic control, the protocol focused on objective surrogate markers like average glucose levels to assess effectiveness. Measuring outcomes would have improved the research design however, due to time constraints, the small sample size, and the lack of a method for measuring outcomes like wound healing, these assessments were not performed.

Results

Forty-four patients were evaluated during the 4-month pilot period including 24 standard care and 20 protocol patients. Admitting diagnoses were similar for both groups with wound care being the most common diagnosis, followed by other infections (urinary tract infection, sepsis, pneumonia) and diabetic ketoacidosis. There was no difference in age, sex, body mass index, HbA1C, or length of stay.

Use of a standardized subcutaneous insulin protocol improved glycemic control over standard care. Blood glucose levels were in range (Mean Blood Glucose [BG] 70–160 mg/dL) for 44.4% of patients on the protocol, versus 30.8% of patients treated with standard care (p<0.05) (Table 7.2).

A common concern of providers and supportive staff is that aggressive glycemic control leads to dangerous low blood sugars. However, in this project there was no difference in hypoglycemic events between standard care and the protocol. Analysis of hypoglycemic events illustrated that the "stacking effects" of regular insulin led to hypoglycemia in both groups. The stacking effect of regular insulin is caused by the onset of action of approximately 30 minutes, and a variable dura-

Table 7.2. Results of Subcutaneous Insulin Protocol			
Variable	**Standard Care**	**Protocol**	**p-value**
Mean blood glucose (BG) (mg/dL)	200	173	<0.05
Mean BG at discharge	175	155	ns[b]
"In-range" 70–160 mg/dL	30.8%	44.4%	<0.05
BG <70 mg/dL (pt. with ≥1 episode)	10	7	ns[b]
Adherence to inpatient guidelines[a]	63.3%	84%	<0.05

[a]American Healthways Inpatient management guidelines for people with diabetes.[7]
[b]ns= not (statistically) significant.

tion of effect that can last 4–6 hours. This variable duration of effect means that the full effects of regular insulin given at breakfast may not be seen by lunchtime. Patient may still have an elevated blood glucose before lunch and be given regular insulin for the meal and to correct the higher than desired blood sugar even though the full effects of the morning dose have not been reached. Thus, this dosing schedule can lead to low, mid-afternoon blood sugars as the cumulative effects of regular insulin from breakfast and lunch coincide. Using ultra-short acting insulin, such as lispro, can alleviate this problem, albeit at a higher financial cost.

For study patients on the protocol, the average blood glucose over the entire hospital stay was almost 30 mg/dL better than those patients receiving standard care. This difference would equate to a 1% decrease in HbA1C if maintained for 3 months. Blood glucose control continued to be better in the protocol group at discharge but was not statistically significant, relative to the comparison group. Increased adherence to inpatient diabetes management guidelines was seen with the protocol versus standard care.

Discussion

Various factors impacted the effectiveness of the protocol, including the ability to predict initial insulin needs, maintenance of consistent dietary intake, patient activity level, and improvement in health. Use of the insulin protocol described in this chapter was equally safe and more effective than standard care for patients in this small pilot study.

Inpatient diabetes management guidelines recommend including lipid profiles, HbA1C, urinary analysis, microalbumin, and electrocardiogram as baseline evaluations upon admission.[11] This project demonstrated that a preprinted protocol could improve the implementation of these guidelines. In the public health system inpatient and outpatient services are commonly provided by the same facility. Therefore, data from the guidelines' recommended baseline evaluations on a particular inpatient admission are readily available for use by that patient's outpatient healthcare providers immediately upon discharge, increasing the continuity of care. This coordination of services helps to provide seamless care for patients and minimizes delays in treatment and followup interventions. This is a different paradigm from many healthcare systems that are not able to coordinate their care between inpatient and outpatient services. Preventative healthcare in a cohort of patients that only seek care from one facility (a captive audience) can reduce costs and morbidities.

Project Updates

Unfortunately, there was insufficient staffing to manage and maintain the protocol beyond this resident's tenure. There was also a change in the internal medicine staff, with over half of the physicians involved in the project no longer providing inpatient services. There is currently no formal interdisciplinary diabetes management team at PIMC, and current glycemic control is based on provider intuition and experience alone.

One lasting effect of the project has been implementation of standing hypoglycemia treatment orders. The hypoglycemia protocol was based on the results and evaluation of this project. Additionally, lessons learned from the project altered the use of short-acting insulin at PIMC. Specifically, since a stacking effect was seen with regular insulin, lispro use has now increased in the inpatient and outpatient settings at PIMC. Previously, the medical center's lispro use was limited secondary to increased cost and no proven benefits over regular insulin.

Topic Updates

Since this project was completed, there have been several articles published on the relative merits of SSI and basal insulin administration. Since patient safety is PIMC's biggest concern, the description of other facilities' insulin use protocols and these protocols' strengths and weaknesses is very useful.[12,13] The development of standing orders, protocols, and use of "best practices" models can be ways to provide excellent diabetes care while improving patient safety.[8,9]

Ultimately, evidence is mounting against short-acting insulin given as sliding scale intermittently and as monotherapy. Most studies are finding that intermittent SSI results in increased hyperglycemic events (and possibly more medical complications) in various patient populations.[4,14,15] The risk of hypoglycemia from SSI varies, and data are not consistent on whether SSI versus other diabetes treatment is more causative, although most studies have not found a statistically significant difference.[14,16-18] Glycemic control is an area where healthcare providers must be vigilant, and the development of a hypoglycemia treatment protocol can help prevent delays in the treatment of events. Several sources have determined that the provision of basal insulin with bolus corrections (similar to PIMC's project) can significantly improve glycemic control, compared to sliding scale insulin alone, for various patient groups.[16,17,19] Pharmacists are in a unique position to change the current trends and thinking of other providers simply by educating them. Showing these providers existing protocols and clinical trial support for using basal plus correction insulin injections, along with the mounting evidence against using sliding scale insulin alone, can help sway providers to change their practices. Persistence is key, along with emphasizing the patient safety concerns that are the root of the Joint Commission's goals.

References

1. UpToDate Online v.15.2 [database online]. *General Principles of Insulin Therapy in Diabetes Mellitus.* Waltham, MA. Updated March 8, 2007.

2. Institute for Healthcare Improvement. Sliding scale insulin protocol. Available at: http://www.ihi.org/IHI/Topics/PatientSafety/MedicationSystems/Tools/SlidingScaleInsulinProtocol.htm. Accessed August 15, 2007.

3. American College of Endocrinology Task Force. Position statement on inpatient diabetes and metabolic control. *Endocr Pract.* 2004;10(1):77-82.

4. Queale WS, Alexander JS, Brancati FL. Glycemic control and sliding scale insulin use in medical inpatients with diabetes mellitus. *Arch Intern Med.* 1997;157:545-552.

5. Gadaleta D, Risucci DA, Nelson RL, et al. Effects of morbid obesity and diabetes mellitus on risk of coronary artery bypass grafting. *Am J Cardiol*. 1992;70:1613-1614.

6. Furnary AP, Zerr KJ, Grunkemeier GL, et al. Continuous intravenous insulin infusion reduces the incidence of deep sternal wound infection in diabetic patients after cardiac surgical procedures. *Ann Thorac Surg*. 1999;67:352-362.

7. Department of Health and Human Services. Diabetes in American Indians and Alaska Natives: Facts At-a-Glance. June 2007. Available at: http://www.ihs.gov/MedicalPrograms/Diabetes. Accessed August 19, 2007.

8. Koproski J, Pretto Z, Poretsky L. Effects of an intervention by a diabetes team in hospitalized patients with diabetes. *Diabetes Care*. 1997;20:1553-1555.

9. Levetan CS, Salas JR, Wilets IF, et al. Impact of endocrine and diabetes team consultation on hospital length of stay for patients with diabetes. *Am J Med*. 1995;99:22-28.

10. 2008 National Patient Safety Goals for Critical Access Hospital Programs. The Joint Commission. Available at: http://www.jointcommission.org/PatientSafety/NationalPatientSafety-Goals/08_cah_npsgs.htm. Accessed August 15, 2007.

11. American Healthways. Inpatient management guidelines for people with diabetes. Nashville, TN; 1999. Available at: http://www.americanhealthways.com.

12. Magee MF. Hospital protocols for targeted glycemic control: development, implementation, and models for cost justification. *Am J Health Syst Pharm*. 2007;64(10 suppl 6):S15-S20.

13. Korytkowski M, Dinardo M, Donihi AC, et al. Evolution of a diabetes inpatient safety committee. *Endocr Pract*. 2006;12(suppl 3):91-99.

14. Freedman RJ, Samson SL, Edwards AL, et al. Glycemic control and use of the insulin sliding scale in hospitalized patients with diabetes. *J Healthc Qual*. 2007;29(2):31-37.

15. Becker T, Moldoveanu A, Cukierman T, et al. Clinical outcomes associated with the use of using subcutaneous insulin-by-glucose sliding scales to manage hyperglycemia in hospitalized patients with pneumonia. *Diabetes Res Clin Pract*. 2007;78(3):392-397.

16. Datta S, Qaadir A, Villanueva G, et al. Once-daily insulin glargine versus 6-hour sliding scale regular insulin for control of hyperglycemia after a bariatric surgical procedure: a randomized clinical trial. *Endocr Pract*. 2007;13(3):225-231.

17. Umpierrez GE, Smiley D, Zisman A, et al. Randomized study of basal bolus insulin therapy in the inpatient management of patients with Type 2 diabetes (RABBIT 2 Trial). *Diabetes Care*. 2007;30(9):2181-2186.

18. Golightly LK, Jones MA, Hamamura DH, et al. Management of diabetes mellitus in hospitalized patients: efficiency and effectiveness of sliding-scale insulin therapy. *Pharmacotherapy*. 2006;26(10):1421-1432.

19. Hassan E. Hyperglycemia management in the hospital setting. *Am J Health Syst Pharm*. 2007 May 15;64(10 suppl 6):S9-S14.

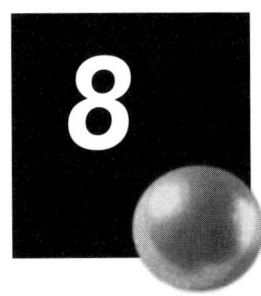

Oh No, She's Got an Insulin Pump! What Do I Do?

Sarah Barber

A young girl is admitted to the emergency department (ED) with a compound fracture of the left tibia, requiring surgery. She also happens to use an insulin pump to manage her insulin dependent diabetes mellitus. The ED physician is concerned about managing her insulin pump, the ED nurse has no idea what to do with the pump, and the surgical resident just exclaimed, "Oh no, she's got an insulin pump! I don't know what to do about that! What do we do?" No one answers the resident. Also, the ED pharmacist isn't really sure how to enter the insulin pump into the pharmacy computer system so accurate dosing information can be documented once the patient is admitted to the floor following surgery.

The Problem

This scenario could happen at any hospital. This wasn't the exact situation that occurred at Children's Hospitals and Clinics of Minnesota, but it was clear that patients with insulin pumps were not receiving optimal care. Once admitted, patients were sometimes unable to continue with their home insulin pump regimen, jeopardizing their ability to keep their blood glucoses in range (less than 120 mg/dL). There were several breakdowns in the system, which led to this suboptimal care during a hospitalization.

Background

Children's Hospitals and Clinics of Minnesota is the sixth largest children's healthcare organization in the United States. It has 326-staffed beds at two hospital campuses in St. Paul and Minneapolis, Minnesota. The health system has state-of-the-art facilities and equipment to meet the special needs of children, with more than half of the beds dedicated to critical care. In 2006, Children's had more than 13,100 admissions, 76,500 emergency room visits, and 119,100 clinic visits with an average of 235 children hospitalized every day. Patient encounters including admissions, surgical procedures, ED and outpatient clinic visits, home care visits, rehab service units, ancillary services, and interpreter services were over 2,027,700 in 2006.[1]

Insulin pumps are small programmable devices about the size of a pager that hold a reservoir of insulin. The pump is programmed to deliver insulin to the body through an infusion set. Patient-administered insulin pumps deliver insulin in a manner designed to mimic the insulin released by a normally functioning pancreas. The endocrinologist and the patient (based on history, glucose levels, food intake, and expected exercise) determine the dosage programmed into the pump. The dosage is designed to match the patient's insulin needs, in both the fasting and fed states. Patients with insulin pumps check their glucose at least four times a day and adjust the insulin pump to maintain near normal glucose values.

At the time the problem with insulin pumps was discovered in June 2004, the institution was participating in Safest in America (SIA), a statewide medication safety action group. The group was specifically looking at insulin safety in hospitals. The hospital SIA insulin team was multidisciplinary, including front line nurses, pharmacists, and nurse managers from a variety of areas, a pharmacy clinical leader, the pharmacy director, and several physicians. The team used opportunity development and planning exercises to determine areas where insulin therapy was problematic. Through this exercise 32 areas (see Table 8.1) for improvement were recognized. Each team member took the list of 32 deficiencies and ranked them based on criticality (how much of an impact fixing this issue would have on insulin safety) and complexity (how difficult the issue would be to fix). Once each area was marked as high, medium, or low in criticality and complexity, each team member then ranked his or her top five of the 32 that needed to be fixed. The team then came back together with this information and determined which areas for improvement would receive the most attention. Several members of the SIA insulin team believed it was important to tackle insulin pump issues because they were becoming such a problem in the health system. A subcommittee was formed to look at insulin pumps, and they also added new members, including a diabetic nurse educator and an ED nurse manager.

The Problem Details

The subcommittee agreed that 1) pharmacists did not consistently enter insulin pump orders into the pharmacy computer system; 2) ED physicians were reluctant to care for patients with insulin pumps because of a lack of knowledge; and 3) nurses were reluctant to make changes in the amount of insulin delivered through the pumps because they just didn't know what to do. When children with insulin pumps were admitted for a nondiabetes-related injury or illness, the nursing staff and physicians (who lacked knowledge about these devices) believed it was safer to discontinue the insulin pumps. As a result, patients' families felt powerless to control their children's diabetes.

Solutions

The committee agreed that changes with insulin pump therapy in the hospital's patients were needed and took the following actions:

- **Insulin Pump History Form and Order Set:** The committee developed order sets in the pharmacy computer system to standardize the way pharmacists enter insulin pump orders. The group also developed an insulin pump history form (Figure 8.1) and written order set (Figure 8.2) to assist with the consistent and accurate ordering of the pump therapy.

- **Algorithms (Decision Trees):** Three separate treatment algorithms were developed for the ED physicians, surgeons, and residents to improve insulin pump safety. These are for hypoglycemia (Figure 8.3), diabetic ketoacidosis (DKA) (Figure 8.4), and nondiabetes-related admissions (Figure 8.5). The algorithms are intended to help physicians make decisions regarding the continuation or discontinuation of the insulin pump. In particular, the hypoglycemia algorithm allows physicians to quickly make a decision to suspend the pump and provide immediate carbohydrates for any hypoglycemic patient with a pump. After stabiliz-

Table 8.1. List of Planning Exercise Areas

Communication/Handoffs

- Orders are confusing
- Orders are not specific enough
- Confusion on who is covering patients especially medical residents chain-of-command
- Off campus consultants—not on site
- Delays in dispensing
- CF diabetes—complication
- Transfer to floor and transition of care
- Medication reconciliation/med history
- Use of abbreviation for insulin type (i.e., "H" for Humalog)

Knowledge and Education

- Lack of familiarity with sliding scale
- Insulin used as complimentary therapy with critical patients
- Confusion about names and types of insulin products
- Different sizes of syringes—TB syringes
- Knowledge base for different types of insulin products
- Lack of centralized database for insulin order, etc.
- Deterioration of knowledge/skill due to patients concentrated on one campus
- Lack of general knowledge about diabetes

Standardization

- Lack of parameter notification and lack of standard order
- Lack of standards for checking blood glucose
- Insulin Pumps: Lack of experience, variations, and parent control. Where is the documentation?
- P.O.C. value vs. serum glucose value—What to use?
- Lack of population specific plans (i.e., Oncology/CF/Surgery)
- Lack of standard concentrations of insulin drips
- Lack of standardized order entry for patients on insulin pumps

Resources

- Lack of P.O.C. testing on Minneapolis campus
- Lack of standards for RN staffing levels

Others

- Look-alike/sound-alike issues
- Wrong patient/wrong drug
- Delays in dietary tray coordination with meals
- Programming IV pumps
- Blood glucose turnaround time
- NPO status glucose monitoring

ing the patient, physicians then determined whether the pump was malfunctioning or if the patient just needed carbohydrates.

The second algorithm, for patients with DKA, also established a quick reference for the physician to determine a course of action for the critically ill patient with an insulin pump. The insulin pump is discontinued only when another form of insulin is available. Finally, the team realized that not all patients with insulin pumps are seen for diabetes-related admissions. Consequently, a nondiabetes-related admission algorithm was developed to make sure that endocrinology was kept in the loop for dosing the insulin pump while the patient was hospitalized. The algorithm would also assist the admitting physician in caring for the patient with an insulin pump.

INSULIN PUMP HISTORY

DATE: _____   TIME: _____

1. **Insulin Pump Brand/Manufacturer/Model Number** _____
2. **Insulin Pump Infusion Set Type** _____
3. **Insulin Pump Settings**
   Basal rates: (List all basal rates)

_____
_____
_____
_____

Food bolus: _____ units/____ gram(s) carbohydrate OR

_____

Correction bolus: ____ units/_____ mg/dL over _____ mg/dL OR
Correction bolus sliding scale:

____ units for blood glucose _____ mg/dL – ___ mg/dL   ____ units for blood glucose _____ mg/dL – ___ mg/dL
____ units for blood glucose _____ mg/dL – ___ mg/dL   ____ units for blood glucose _____ mg/dL – ___ mg/dL
____ units for blood glucose _____ mg/dL – ___ mg/dL   ____ units for blood glucose _____ mg/dL – ___ mg/dL
____ units for blood glucose _____ mg/dL – ___ mg/dL   ____ units for blood glucose _____ mg/dL – ___ mg/dL
____ units for blood glucose _____ mg/dL – ___ mg/dL   ____ units for blood glucose _____ mg/dL – ___ mg/dL

4. **Hypoglycemia**: What are your parameters for treating hypoglycemia?

_____
_____
_____

5. **Lab work:** How often do you check your blood glucose at home? Every ____ hours.

6. **Dose calculator features:** (e.g., Bolus Wizard®).

_____
_____

7. **CDE Assessment of Insulin Pump Support Plan during Hospitalization:**

   a. Download pump in diabetes clinic:_____ (Place download reports in inpatient chart)

   b. Review of current settings: Basal rate: _____ Bolus amounts: _____

   c. Review of safety settings: Max basal rate: _____ Max bolus rate: _____ Alarms: On ___ Off___

   d. Dosage calculator program settings: On_____ Off_____ (Dosage calculator settings: place in chart from download)

   e. Assessment of pump support plan:_____
   _____
   _____

   Signed: _____ RN/CDE

Figure 8.1. Insulin Pump History Form.

- **Nursing Clinical Standard for Insulin Pumps**: The subcommittee recognized during the development of algorithms and order sets that the nursing clinical standard for insulin pumps had been discontinued. The group sought reinstatement of this nursing clinical standard to ensure nursing had a reference/resource for caring for patients with insulin pumps. The standard needed revisions because of the new order forms and algorithms. The group also worked with risk management to ensure the guideline was consistent with applicable legal standards

INSULIN PUMP ORDERS

Date: _____   Time: _____

Weight: _____mg   Allergies: _____

1. **Insulin Pump Brand/Manufacturer/Model Number** _____

2. **Insulin Pump Infusion Set Type**_____

3. **Pharmacy to send insulin for use in pump.** (Select one)

    ☐ Insulin Aspart (Novolog®)   ☐ Other (Please specify) _____

    ☐ Insulin Lispro (Humalog®)

4.   Pharmacy to enter the following parameters for medication administration record

  ☑ **Basal rates**: (List all basal rates)

  _____

  _____

  _____

  _____

  _____

  ☑ **Food bolus**: _____ units/____ gram(s) carbohydrate OR

  _____

  ☐ **Correction bolus**: ____ units/_____ mg/dL over _____ mg/dL OR
  ☐ **Correction bolus sliding scale** :

_____ units for blood glucose _____ mg/dL – ____mg/dL	_____ units for blood glucose _____ mg/dL – _____ mg/dL
_____ units for blood glucose _____ mg/dL – ____mg/dL	_____ units for blood glucose _____ mg/dL – _____ mg/dL
_____ units for blood glucose _____ mg/dL – ____mg/dL	_____ units for blood glucose _____ mg/dL – _____ mg/dL
_____ units for blood glucose _____ mg/dL – ____mg/dL	_____ units for blood glucose _____ mg/dL – _____ mg/dL
_____ units for blood glucose _____ mg/dL – ____mg/dL	_____ units for blood glucose _____ mg/dL – _____ mg/dL

  Call HO or attending MD for blood glucose greater than (>) _____ mg/dL or less than(<) _____ mg/dL

5. **Hypoglycemia**: Treat per nursing clinical standard (treatment of hypoglycemia in children with diabetes) and using the hypoglycemia decision tree for insulin pump.

6. **Lab Work**

  ☐ Postoperative patient

    ☐ Check point-of-care blood glucose every 2 hr for ____ hours postoperatively

    ☐ Consult physician of record or surgeon for blood glucose greater than (>) 250 mg/dL

  ☐ Other patients (Non-postoperative)

    ☐ Check point-of-care blood glucose every _____ hr.

    ☐ Consult physician of record or surgeon for blood glucose greater than (>) 400 mg/dL

7. **Other Orders**

  ☐ Discontinue dose calculator feature of pump (e.g., Bolus Wizard®).

  ☐ Consult endocrinologist (for dosing)

  ☐ Consult clinical diabetic educator (for assistance restarting pump)

_____MD

Figure 8.2. Insulin Order Set.

so patients and their families could continue to manage their insulin pump and their diabetes once hospitalized.

- **Education:** The group, working with clinical nurse educators, used nursing education days to teach nurses more about insulin pumps and improve their comfort with helping fami-

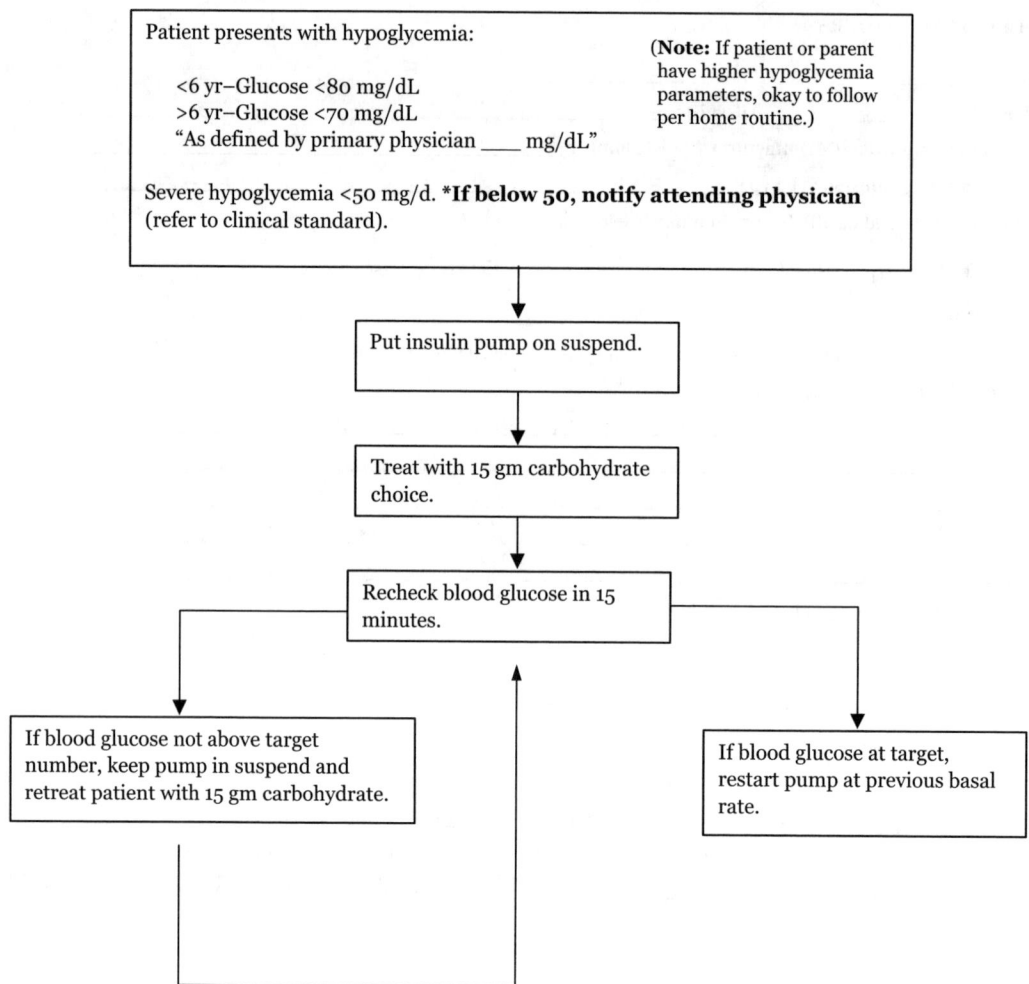

Figure 8.3. Hypoglycemia Decision Tree.

lies make changes; and improved documentation on the medication administration record (MAR) and diabetic flowchart. This training provided hands-on experience with the pumps and first time views of the order forms and documentation changes. A single medical/surgical unit on the St. Paul campus was most affected by these policy changes, because most of the patients utilizing insulin pumps in St. Paul would be on this unit.

The group's ultimate goal was to empower families to assist with their child's diabetes care while the child was hospitalized.

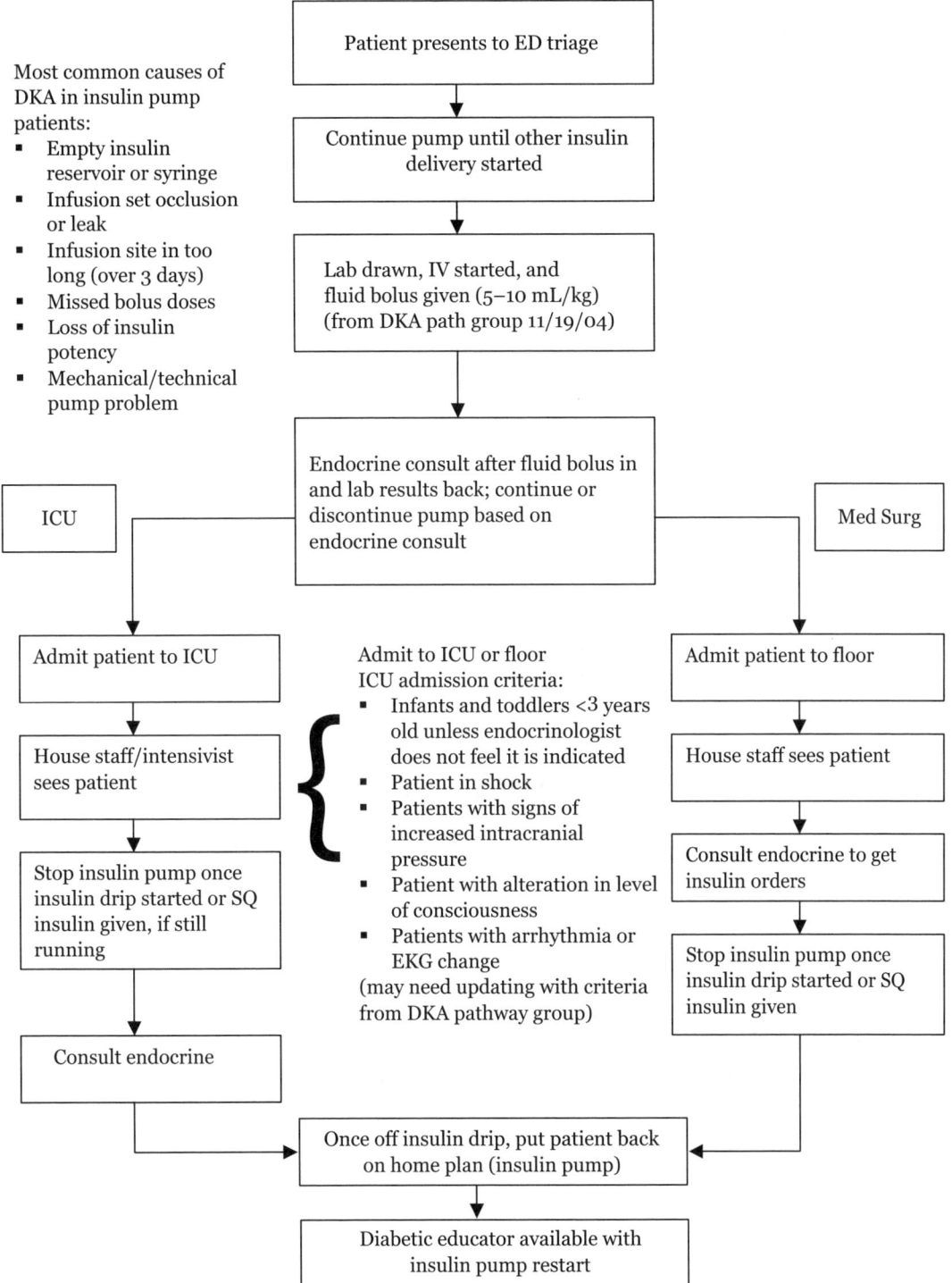

Figure 8.4. DKA Decision Tree.

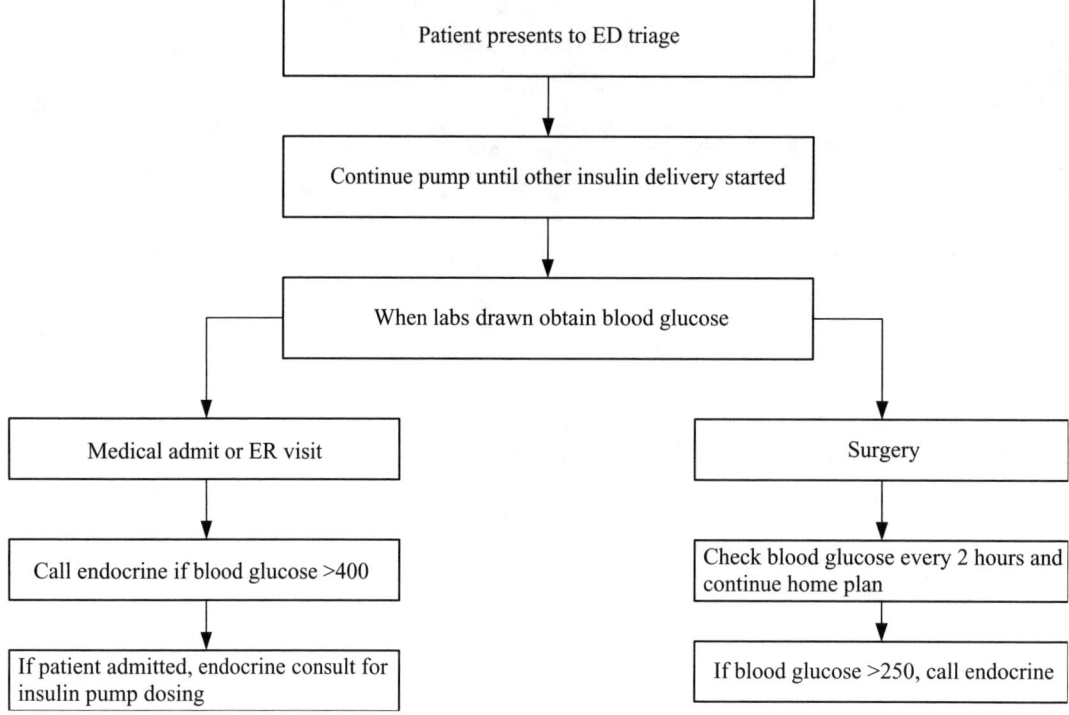

Figure 8.5. ED Visit/Medical/Surgical Admission (nondiabetes related).

Implementation and Results

The full changes were implemented after the education days in November of 2005. In September 2006, the hospital changed from computerized paper medication administration records (MARs) to electronic medication administration records (eMARs) and electronic medical record (EMR) documentation. This presented new challenges and prompted updates to the order sets based on the EMR documentation and appearance of the orders on the eMAR.

The subcommittee believes that these changes have improved the care of patients with insulin pumps. This is a high risk, low volume problem. In the first year after implementation from November 2005 to December 2006, six patients with insulin pumps were admitted for non-DKA or restarts after DKA, with one patient admitted through the ED. Pharmacists are now consistently entering orders using the predefined order set and enforcing the use of the order forms by physicians. The ED physicians feel comfortable using the algorithm to continue insulin pump therapy. The nurses feel much more comfortable using the pumps and patients' families feel that they are empowered to care for their children's diabetes. Recently, a surgical patient with an insulin pump was able to continue her home regimen and all blood glucose tests while hospitalized were within her goal range of less than 100 mg/dL.

Since the implementation of the order sets, insulin pump history, the algorithms, and other resources, Children's Hospitals and Clinics of Minnesota has also implemented an EMR and eMAR. Implementation of the EMR has forced changes to the insulin pump forms and computer order sets developed by the committee (Figure 8.6). Insulin pump therapy in the hospital will continue to be an evolving process and the hospital will continue to have more hospitalized patients with insulin pumps as the use of the insulin pump continues to grow. The next time you see a patient

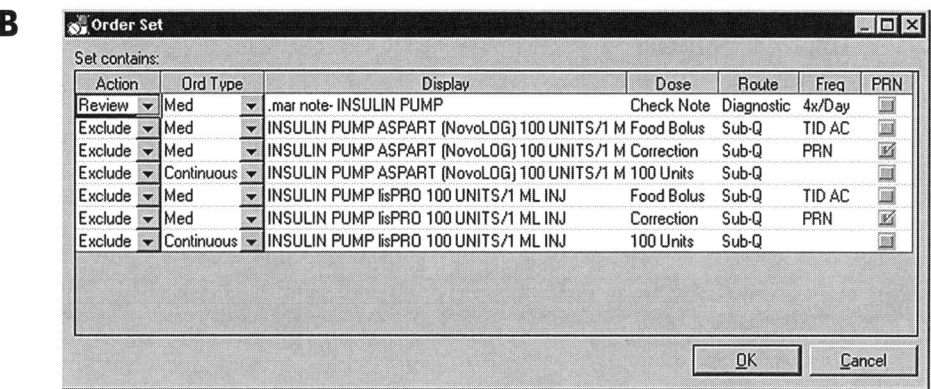

Figure 8.6. A) Computerized Order Set for Pharmacists in the Pharmacy Informatics System, Original Order Set (prior to implementation of eMAR). B) Current State Order Set (postimplementation of eMAR).

with an insulin pump, don't panic! Instead take steps now to empower patients and their families to continue to self-manage their diabetes.

Reference

1. http://www.childrensmn.org/Communities/AboutUs.asp.

Resources

American Diabetes Association, Clinical Practice Recommendations 2003. Continuous subcutaneous insulin infusion. *Diabetes Care.* 2003;26(suppl 1):S125.

ASHP Section of Inpatient Care Practitioners. Professional Practice Recommendations for Safe Use of Insulin in Hospitals. ASHP. Available at: www.ashp.org. Accessed October 2006. Also available at: www.ashp.org/emplibrary/Safe_Use_of_Insulin.pdf. Portions reprinted in *Pharmacy Insider*, Fall 2006.

Medtronic. Guidelines for the Hospitalized Pump Patient. 2004.

Metchick L, Petit W, Inzucchi S. Inpatient management of diabetes mellitus. *Am J Med.* 2002;113(4):317-323.

Stephens E, Riddle M. Evolving approaches to intensive insulin therapy in type I diabetes: multiple daily injections, insulin pumps and new methods of monitoring. *Rev Endocr Metab Disord.* 2003;4(4):325-334.

Willi S, Planton J, Egede L, et al. Benefits of continuous subcutaneous insulin infusion in children with Type I diabetes. *J Pediatr.* 2003;143(6):796-801.

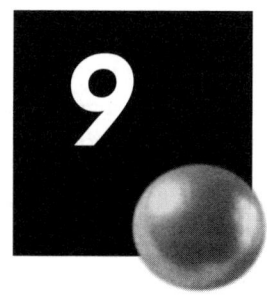

Strategies to Enhance Tobacco Cessation Education in Your Hospital

Alan J. Zillich

Frank Vitale

Karen Suchanek Hudmon

Introduction

Cigarette smoking is the leading cause of morbidity and mortality in the United States, contributing to the deaths of nearly 440,000 Americans each year.[1] Smoking causes many diseases by harming nearly every organ of the body, negatively impacting individuals at all stages of life—unborn babies, infants, children, adolescents, adults, and seniors.[2] Compared to nonsmokers, adults who smoke are more likely to be hospitalized and suffer hospital-related complications (e.g., postoperative infections, delayed wound healing, respiratory infections).[3,4] These complications can be reduced if patients quit smoking, and the hospital provides an ideal setting and opportunity to initiate smoking cessation.

During a hospital admission, a "teachable moment" is created.[5] The patient may be motivated to make a behavioral change as a result of their hospital admission and the salient nature of their disease. The patient is also captive in a setting where smoking is prohibited, and the most severe withdrawal symptoms occur during the first 2–3 days of the admission. Two published meta-analyses concluded that intensive inpatient smoking cessation programs are highly effective.[6,7] In one program, the proportion of patients who remained abstinent from smoking at 3 and 12 months approached 50%.[8]

Strategies to facilitate smoking cessation education within the hospital setting are needed, because there are large gaps between the knowledge of cessation interventions and widespread adoption and implementation of these interventions.[9] National assessments conducted in 2001 indicate that a median of 43% of Medicare beneficiary inpatients receive smoking cessation counseling during hospitalization.[10] Smoking cessation education is a reportable performance measure from the the Joint Commission™.[11] As this quality care indicator becomes linked to reimbursement, hospitals and healthcare facilities need strategies to enable compliance with indicators associated with the delivery of smoking cessation education to patients who smoke. The purpose of this chapter is to outline several strategies that may be useful in achieving this goal.

Intervention Strategies

A variety of strategies can be used to enhance delivery of smoking cessation education to hospitalized patients. The pages that follow delineate a compilation of strategies used from several hospital systems, most notably, Wishard Health System in Indianapolis, IN. Wishard is a large, tax-supported, urban teaching public healthcare system that cares for a large number of medically uninsured and underinsured via a university medical center. The health system includes a 350-bed hospital, emergency department, on-site ambulatory care services, and a network of community health centers located throughout the city. Four strategies are discussed: (1) education of professional staff; (2) promotion of tobacco cessation resources for patients; (3) a counseling algorithm for delivery of smoking cessation education to patients; and (4) development of an order form for tobacco dependence treatment.

Education of Professional Staff

Although most patients interact with multiple healthcare providers during their inpatient stay, the acute nature of the hospitalization often limits the time and extent of cessation education that any one healthcare professional can deliver. Because the U.S. Public Health Service *Clinical Practice Guideline for Treating Tobacco Use and Dependence* recommends that *all* healthcare providers offer brief, smoking cessation education and because patients who receive cessation advice from multiple providers are more likely to quit than are patients who receive cessation advice from one provider,[5] all clinicians in the health system should participate in a tobacco cessation training program, and all clinicians should promote cessation (and document activities) at each possible contact with a given patient.

To the extent possible, the education should follow recommendations from the *Clinical Practice Guideline*, which advocates a "5 A's" framework for comprehensive tobacco cessation counseling: (1) **A**sk about tobacco use; (2) **A**dvise patients to quit; (3) **A**ssess readiness to quit; (4) **A**ssist with quitting; and (5) **A**rrange followup care.[5] In the hospital setting, it is not expected that one clinician would provide all of the five elements of cessation counseling—instead, clinicians who are in contact with the patient during hospitalization should integrate an Ask-Advise-Refer protocol as part of a clinical encounter with each patient. Through the referral process, the Assess-Assist-Arrange components can be addressed. Training materials for the Ask-Advise-Refer model are available for free at www.ashp.org/tobacco and rxforchange.ucsf.edu. The following steps for adoption of the Ask-Advise-Refer model are delineated:

- **Ask:** The first step in providing tobacco cessation education is to identify all tobacco users. Tobacco use status (current, former quit in past 12 months, former quit more than 12 months ago, never) should be documented in the medical record. The Ask component should be embedded within the admission process. Include the question "Have you smoked or used any type of tobacco in the past month?" on the admission form, and if the patient indicates "yes" then assess the amount of tobacco used (current tobacco users) or the date of the last use (former tobacco users).

- **Advise:** Healthcare providers should advise all tobacco users to quit. The advice should be clear, strong, personalized, and conveyed in a tone emphasizing concern for the patient's health and a commitment to help them with quitting. Messages can be personalized by linking the importance of quitting to the individual's current health status. Consider using the following two phrases. (1) "Quitting is the single most important thing you can do to improve your health now and in the future. I strongly recommend that you quit as soon as possible, and I can help." (2) "I see from your chart that you smoked prior to your hospitalization. Because of the bans on smoking in the hospital, it has probably been difficult for you not to smoke since you've been here. I hope you will take this opportunity to consider yourself an ex-smoker, and I can help you with the process of quitting for good."[9]

- **Refer:** Quitting tobacco is best approached with a multicomponent treatment plan involving drug therapy in conjunction with behavioral counseling. While medications can quickly be prescribed during a patient's hospital stay, behavioral therapy can require significant time commitment for clinicians. In the absence of time or expertise for providing comprehensive behavioral counseling, patients should be referred to other resources. The referral process should be aided by a patient handout containing information about resources for quitting.

Promotion of Tobacco Cessation Resources

Telephone quitlines are a primary resource to refer patients for help with the quitting process. Quitlines provide one-on-one counseling, self-help kits, and individualized cessation information at no charge to the patient. The quitline is available during and after the hospital admission to ensure continuity of care. The following phrase can be used by clinicians to provide referrals: "Consider calling the national quitline number, 1-800-QUIT-NOW. Smoking cessation specialists will give you personalized help, by telephone, at no cost during and after your hospital stay." Studies have shown that patients who receive quitline counseling are twice as likely to quit compared with patients who quit on their own.[12]

As an alternative to telephone quitlines, patients can be referred to local tobacco cessation programs or Web-based programs (see Resources). Organizations such as health departments, healthcare facilities, and local chapters of the American Lung Association may offer smoking cessation programs. Contact your local health department to help identify local resources. Finally, patients can be referred to Internet resources such as www.quitnet.com. The Wishard hospital pharmacy developed a one-page handout for patients to promote various tobacco cessation resources (see Figure 9.1). Hospital staff have used the phrase "Here's a list of smoking cessation resources to help you quit. Let's review the list and discuss what might be best for you."

Counseling Algorithm for Tobacco Cessation

The rationale for creating a counseling algorithm was threefold. First, the algorithm guided clinicians through the Ask-Advise-Refer protocol. Second, the algorithm functioned as a documentation tool for any clinician to quickly document tobacco cessation counseling activities for each patient. Third, the tool served as a uniform data source for retrospective examination of tobacco cessation education compliance with Joint Commission mandates. With collaboration from information technology personnel, the algorithm was developed to interface with the hospital's electronic medical record (Figure 9.2). However, the questions on the tool could easily be adapted to other healthcare facilities for use in providing and documenting tobacco cessation counseling.

Each patient encounter is entered into the patients' electronic medical record using the algorithm. Furthermore, patients who indicate that they are willing to quit smoking are asked if they can be contacted by a representative of the health system's tobacco cessation program. This representative will contact the patient, generally before discharge, and ask if they are interested in enrolling in the cessation program. This program, supported by state and county funding, is a series of three group classes that focus on behavior modification. Pharmacotherapy is provided at low cost.

Treatment Order Form for Tobacco Dependence

Given that tobacco is the primary preventable cause of disease and death in the U.S., it is a primary cause of hospitalizations. As such, all hospitals systems should have well-established tobacco dependence treatment protocols in place, and compliance with this protocol should approach 100%. In congruence with recommendations set forth in the *Clinical Practice Guideline for Treating Tobacco Use and Dependence*,[5] the protocol should combine both FDA-approved medications for smoking cessation and behavioral counseling. A first step is to examine the smoking cessation medications

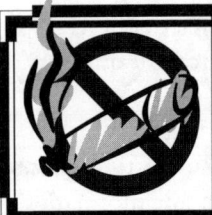 # THINKING ABOUT QUITTING?

Here are some **things to do** while you consider quitting:

- Write down your reasons to quit smoking.
- Write down your concerns about quitting. Think of ways to relieve your concerns.
- Ask your family and friends for support while you are quitting.
- Think about situations when you would be tempted to smoke. Plan ways to cope with these situations.

Did you know that there are programs and treatments available to help you quit?

For more information:
- Talk to your doctor or pharmacist about medicines to help you quit.
- Call Wishard Health Services at (317) 287-3717
- Go the internet site http://www.quitnet.com
- Call the toll free tobacco quit line 800-QUIT-NOW

Figure 9.1. Patient Education Sheet.

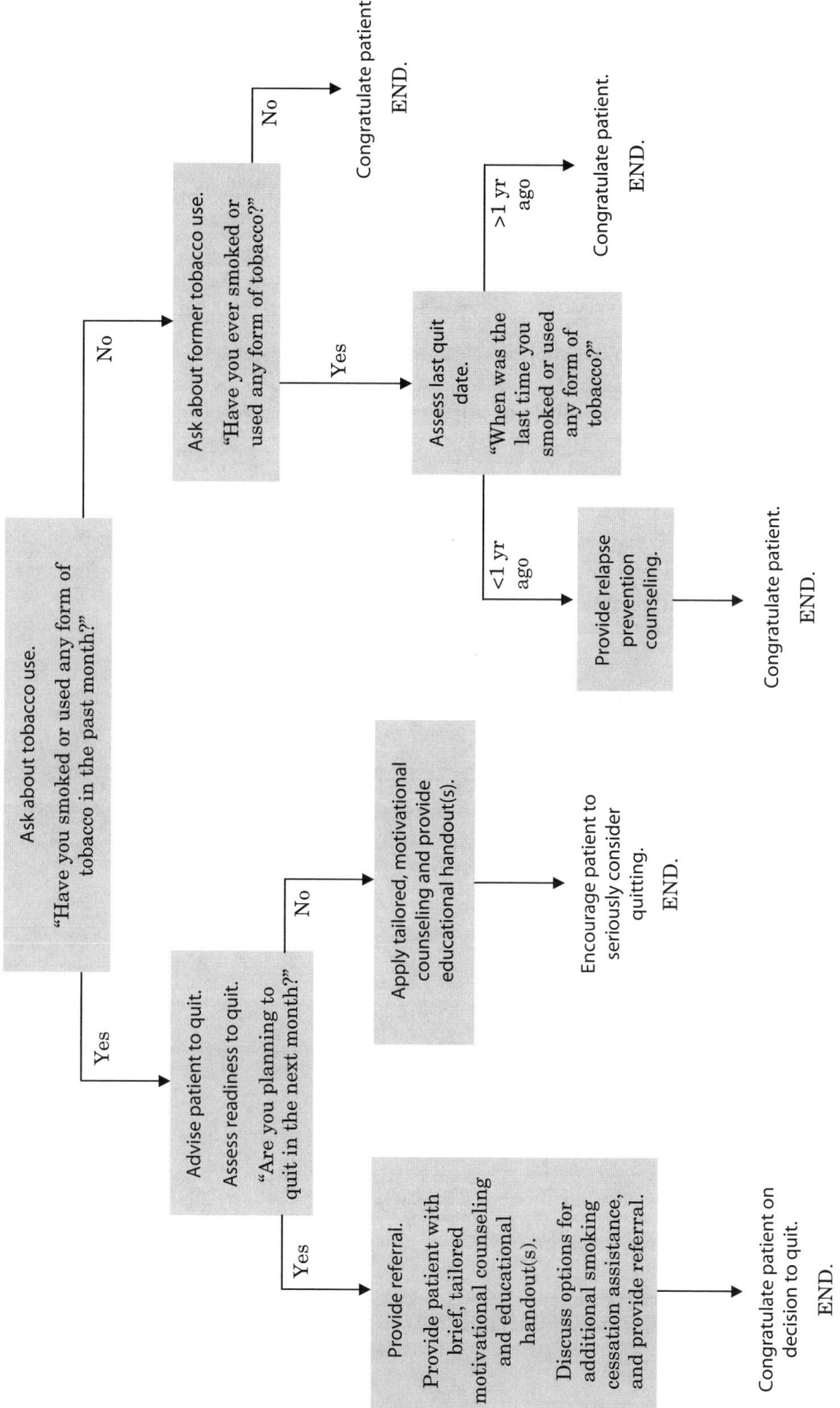

Figure 9.2. Counseling Algorithm.

available on the hospital formulary. Formularies should include one long-acting (transdermal patch) and several short-acting (gum, lozenge, oral inhaler, nasal spray) nicotine dosage formulation, as well as bupropion SR and varenicline. These options provide a range of therapeutic options. Figure 9.3 contains a sample Tobacco Dependence Treatment Order Form, which delineates a straightforward, yet comprehensive approach to provision of tobacco cessation services. A copy of this form should reside in the patients' chart throughout the hospital stay. Discharge orders should also be documented on the form. If applicable for your institution, include a plan for outpatient followup contact at 1 week and 1 month.

Summary

The information presented in this chapter reflects a combination of strategies that should be used to enhance tobacco cessation education in your hospital. These strategies incorporate lessons learned during development and implementation. All patients must be asked about tobacco use on intake, and this assessment should characterize the type and amount of tobacco used for current users, as well as the date of last use for former tobacco users. All clinicians who come into contact with a patient should strongly advise the patient to quit, and all patients who have used any form of tobacco in the past year should receive counseling. Current smokers should be initiated on FDA-approved medications for smoking cessation, except when medically contraindicated, and discharge orders for medication and additional behavioral counseling should be provided.

Resources

American Cancer Society
800-ACS-2345 or www.cancer.org

American Heart Association
800-242-8721 or www.americanheart.org

American Legacy Foundation
202-454-5555 or www.americanlegacy.org

American Lung Association
800-LUNG-USA or www.lungusa.org

Centers for Disease Control and Prevention
800-311-3435 or www.cdc.gov/tobacco

Rx for Change: Clinician-Assisted Tobacco Cessation
rxforchange.ucsf.edu

Product-Specific Programs
www.nicorette.com, www.commitlozenge.com, www.nicodermcq.com, www.nicotrol.com, www.committedquitters.com, www.zyban.com, www.chantix.com, www.get-quit.com

Telephone Quitlines
1-800-QUIT-NOW or www.smokefree.gov/talk.html

Tobacco Dependence Treatment Order Form

Date: _____ Time: _____ | Patient Imprint

Medication (for current smokers): *Refer to Package Insert for Complete Usage Instructions*

Nicotine Patch

☐ <10 cigarettes/day: 14 mg patch. Replace patch every 24 hours. Rotate application site.

☐ ≥10 cigarettes/day: 21 mg patch. Replace patch every 24 hours. Rotate application site.

Nicotine Gum

☐ <25 cigarettes/day: 2 mg gum, 1 piece every 1–2 hours while awake. Patient must **activate** gum by chewing slowly until peppery/tingling sensation appears, then **park** between cheek and gums until sensation disappears. Reactivate gum by chewing slowly until sensation reappears, then re-park. Gum should be removed after 30 minutes.

☐ ≥25 cigarettes/day: 4 mg gum, 1 piece every 1–2 hours while awake. Patient must **activate** gum by chewing slowly until peppery/tingling sensation appears, then **park** between cheek and gums until sensation disappears. Reactivate gum by chewing slowly until sensation reappears, then re-park. Gum should be removed after 30 minutes.

Nicotine Lozenge

☐ First cigarette >30 minutes after waking: 2 mg lozenge, 1 lozenge every 1–2 hours while awake. Patient should use like a cough drop. Do not chew or swallow.

☐ First cigarette ≤30 minutes after waking: 4 mg lozenge, 1 lozenge every 1–2 hours while awake. Patient should use like a cough drop. Do not chew or swallow.

Bupropion SR tablets

☐ 150 mg QD for 3 days, then 150 mg BID

Varenicline tablets

☐ 0.5 mg QD for 3 days, then 0.5 mg BID for 4 days, then 1 mg BID

Inpatient Education (for current smokers and smokers who quit <12 months ago):

☐ Provide counseling to this patient on cessation

☐ Provide patient with education materials and resources

Discharge and Followup (for current smokers and smokers who quit <12 months ago):

☐ Refer patient to_____ for additional assistance

☐ Provide patient with discharge prescription for cessation medication

Physician/Provider Signature:_____

Check if applicable:

☐ Patient refused treatment

☐ Neurological deficits preclude counseling

☐ Physical/mental status prevents patient from smoking

Figure 9.3. Tobacco Cessation Order Form.

Clinical Practice Guideline Materials
U.S. Department of Health and Human Services
http://www.surgeongeneral.gov/tobacco/
Publications Clearinghouse
P.O. Box 8547
Silver Spring, MD 20907
1-800-358-9295

Web-Based Programs for Quitting
www.quitnet.com, www.way2quit.com, www.mytimetoquit.com

Other Informational Web Sites
smokingcessationleadership.ucsf.edu, www.tobaccofreenurses.org, www.ashp.org/tobacco

Check with your local health department to identify specific programs in your area.

References

1. Annual smoking-attributable mortality, years of potential life lost, and productivity losses—United States, 1997–2001. *MMWR Morb Mortal Wkly Rep.* 2005;54:625-628.

2. U.S. Department of Health and Human Services. *The Health Consequences of Smoking: A Report of the Surgeon General.* Washington, DC: U.S. Department of Health and Human Services, Centers for Disease Control and Prevention, National Center for Chronic Disease Prevention and Health Promotion, Office on Smoking and Health; 2004.

3. Egan TD, Wong KC. Perioperative smoking cessation and anesthesia: a review. *J Clin Anesth.* 1992;4:63-72.

4. Hodgson TA. Cigarette smoking and lifetime medical expenditures. *Milbank Q.* 1992;70:81-125.

5. U.S. Department of Health and Human Services. *Treating Tobacco Use and Dependence, Clinical Practice Guideline.* Rockville, MD: U.S. Public Health Service; 2000.

6. France EK, Glasgow RE, Marcus AC. Smoking cessation interventions among hospitalized patients: what have we learned? *Prev Med.* 2001;32:376-388.

7. Rigotti NA, Munafo MR, Murphy MF, et al. Interventions for smoking cessation in hospitalized patients. *Cochrane Database Syst Rev.* 2003(1):CD001837.

8. Stevens VJ, Glasgow RE, Hollis JF, et al. A smoking-cessation intervention for hospital patients. *Med Care.* 1993;31:65-72.

9. Smith PM, Taylor CB. *Implementing an Inpatient Smoking Cessation Program.* 1st ed. Mahwah, NJ: Lawrence Erlbaum Assoc; 2006.

10. Jencks SF, Huff ED, Cuerdon T. Change in the quality of care delivered to Medicare beneficiaries, 1998–1999 to 2000–2001. *JAMA.* 2003;289:305-312.

11. Centers for Medicare and Medicaid Services (CMS). *Specifications manual for national hospital quality measures, version 1.04.* Washington, DC: Centers for Medicare and Medicaid Services, The Joint Commission on Accreditation of Healthcare Organizations (JCAHO); 2005.

12. Zhu SH, Anderson CM, Tedeschi GJ, et al. Evidence of real-world effectiveness of a telephone quitline for smokers. *N Engl J Med.* 2002;347:1087-1093.

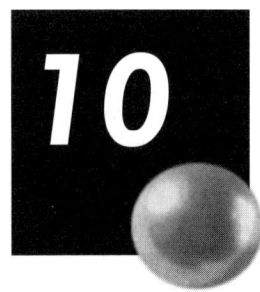

Is My Patient Pregnant? Is My Patient Lactating?

Antonia Alafris

Henry Cohen

Acknowledgments: The authors would like to recognize the contributions of Nympha Meindel, RN, Stacey Lutz, Angela Belfer, RN, Gargi Sethi, MS, John Tierney, Argy Chafouleas, RN, and E. Zoed Matos. Each person is affiliated with Kingsbrook Jewish Medical Center, with the exception of Zoed Matos, who is affiliated with Z-Consulting, LLC, Meriden, Connecticut.

Background

Kingsbrook Jewish Medical Center (KJMC) was founded in 1925 as a private, not-for-profit institution. It has 864 beds with 326 in the acute care hospital and 538 in the long-term care facility, Rutland Nursing Home. The technology currently available on the acute care side includes a computerized, physician order-entry system (CPOE; Siemens Invision®); a pharmacy application (Siemens® Pharmacy); an electronic medication administration record (Siemens® MAK); and a robotic system (McKesson® Rx) for dispensing unit-dose packaged medications. A bidirectional interface exists between the CPOE system, the pharmacy application, and MAK. That is, once a physician enters a medication order in the CPOE system, the order interfaces to the pharmacy application and MAK. At that point, the pharmacist reviews the patient's electronic profile (e.g., diagnosis, laboratory findings, concomitant medications) to ensure that the drug, dose, route, and frequency of the new medication order are appropriate for the patient. If everything is appropriate, the pharmacist verifies the medication order. Once the medication order is verified, the nurse can administer the medication to the patient and chart in MAK the date and time that the medication was given.

The Problem

According to the medication management standard 1.10 of the the Joint Commission™, a patient's pregnancy and lactation status must be readily available to all those involved in the medication management of the patient.[1] The administration of the pharmacy, nursing, and medicine departments decided to utilize KJMC's current technology to capture the required data.[1] After a meeting with the assistant directors of the departments of clinical information services, pharmacy, nursing, and medicine, a decision was made that the pregnancy and lactation status of every female patient between the ages of 12 and 50 should be captured and be readily available to all healthcare providers.

The Solution

The team of assistant directors and the senior applications analyst decided that the pregnancy and lactation status should be obtained during the patient's initial assessment, which is completed by the admitting nurse. As a result, two fields were added to the patient initial assessment screen in the CPOE system (Figure 10.1): "Is Pt Pregnant? and "Is Pt Lactating?" The nurse has the option to answer either "Y" for "yes" or "N" for "no."

In addition, the group decided that the pregnancy and lactation status of the patient had to be readily available to the pharmacist and the nurse in MAK. As a result, the senior applications analyst created two extra fields on the header of the pharmacy application and MAK where the pregnancy and lactation status information ("Y" or "N") would interface (Figure 10.2) and be readily available to the pharmacist and the nurse.

A drawback of the present technology is that it does not have the logic to *assess* the pregnancy and lactation status of a patient and alert the physician, pharmacist, or nurse not to prescribe, dispense, or administer a pregnancy category X or D medication. To aid the healthcare professional and protect the patient from being given a pregnancy category X or D medication, the pharmacy administration decided to identify all such medications in the drug master file. With the help of the senior applications analyst, all pregnancy category X or D medications were flagged in the CPOE system. A screen was created by the clinical applications analyst (Figure 10.3) where every time a pregnancy category X or D medication was prescribed—for a female patient between the ages of 12 and 50—the physician would need to check "Yes" or "No" regarding the patient status. If "Yes" or "No" were not checked off, the prescribing process for that pregnancy category X or D medication could not be completed. The answer that the physician chose then interfaced to the directions field for that medication order (Figure 10.4) which then interfaced to the "Add'l Sigs" field in the pharmacy application (Figure 10.5). This way the pharmacist is aware of the pregnancy and lactation

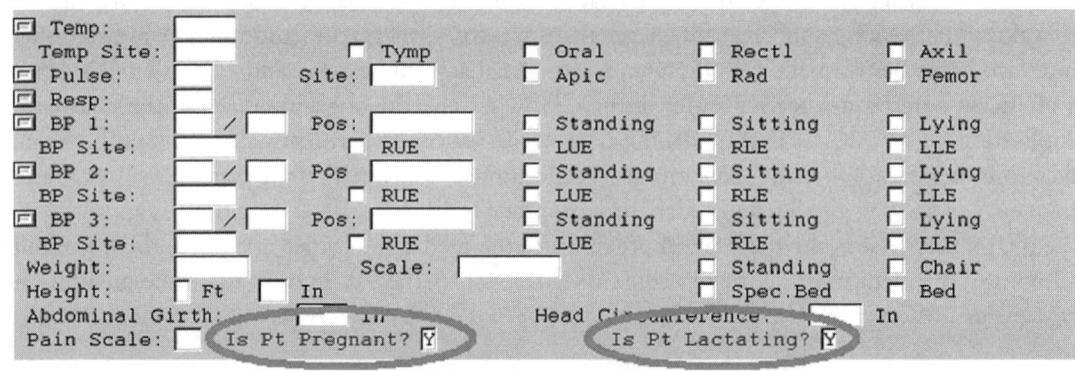

Figure 10.1. Patient Initial Assessment Screen in CPOE System.

PT#: 27401	SEX: F	DOB: 01/01/1964	HT: 5f 5 in
MR#: 11254	SVC: MED	AGE: 42Y	WT: 265 lb
ROOM/BED: B8 807A		ATT DR: XXXXX,	IBW: 59.3 KG
DIAG:		ADM D/T: 07/05/2006 13:40	BSA: 2.428 M2
		LOS: 106	CrCl: N/C ML/MII
ALLERGIES/ADRs:	PCN; CEPH; CARBAP, SALICYLATES; NSAIDS; PYRAZOLES, BETA-ADRENERGI		
PREGNANT? NO			
LACTATING? NO			

Figure 10.2. Header of Patient Profile in the Pharmacy Application and MAK.

status of the patient (in case the information on the header was missed or if the pharmacist was not aware that the prescribed medication was pregnancy category X or D). With the current system, the physician is only alerted that the pregnancy and lactation status of the patient must be confirmed prior to prescribing the drug; it does not stop the physician from ordering the medication if he/she checks off "Yes" regarding the pregnancy and lactation status of the patient. As a result, the physician is able to prescribe a pregnancy category X or D medication to a pregnant or lactating female. In this case, the pharmacist should not verify the medication order and he/she should contact the prescriber to change the medication to a safe alternative.

The pregnancy category of all new medications (formulary or nonformulary) that are added to the drug master file are reviewed by the pharmacy administration. If the drug is pregnancy category X or D, the clinical applications analyst is alerted to ensure that the medication is flagged as such in the CPOE system. However, if the physician orders a medication that is not part of the drug master file and he/she free-texts the drug name in the CPOE system, clinical checking is bypassed and the physician is not alerted to indicate the pregnancy and lactation status of the patient. Once the medication order interfaces to the pharmacy application, it is up to the pharmacist to identify the medication as a pregnancy category X or D drug, contact the physician to learn the pregnancy and lactation status of the patient, and determine whether it is appropriate for the patient to receive the drug. It is the policy of the pharmacy department that all medication orders are comprehensively reviewed by the pharmacist prior to being validated, especially for nonformulary medications with which the pharmacist may be unfamiliar.

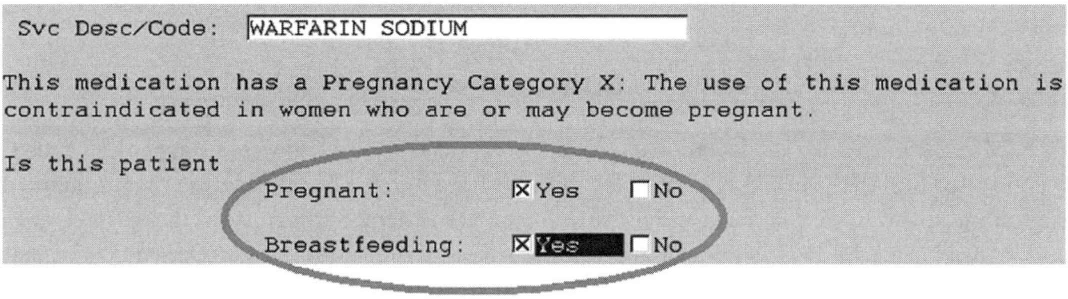

Figure 10.3. Screen in CPOE System Identifying All Pregnancy X or D Medications and Forcing the Prescriber to Identify the Patient's Pregnancy and Lactation Status.

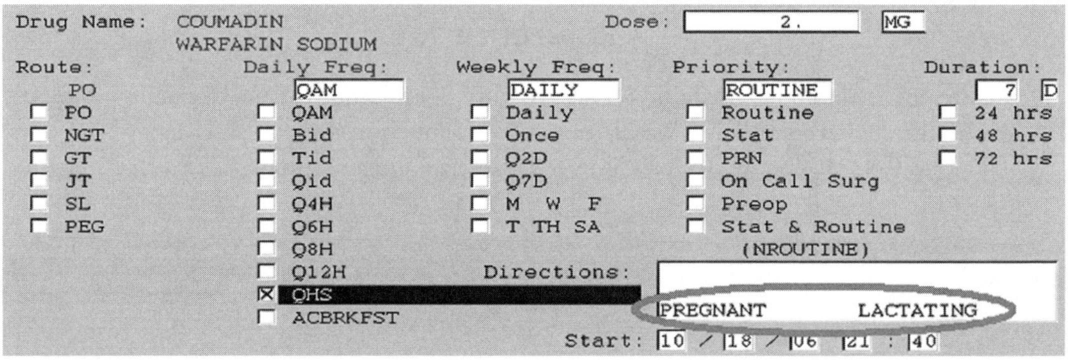

Figure 10.4. The Pregnancy and Lactation Status of the Patient Interfaces to the Directions Field of the Medication Order.

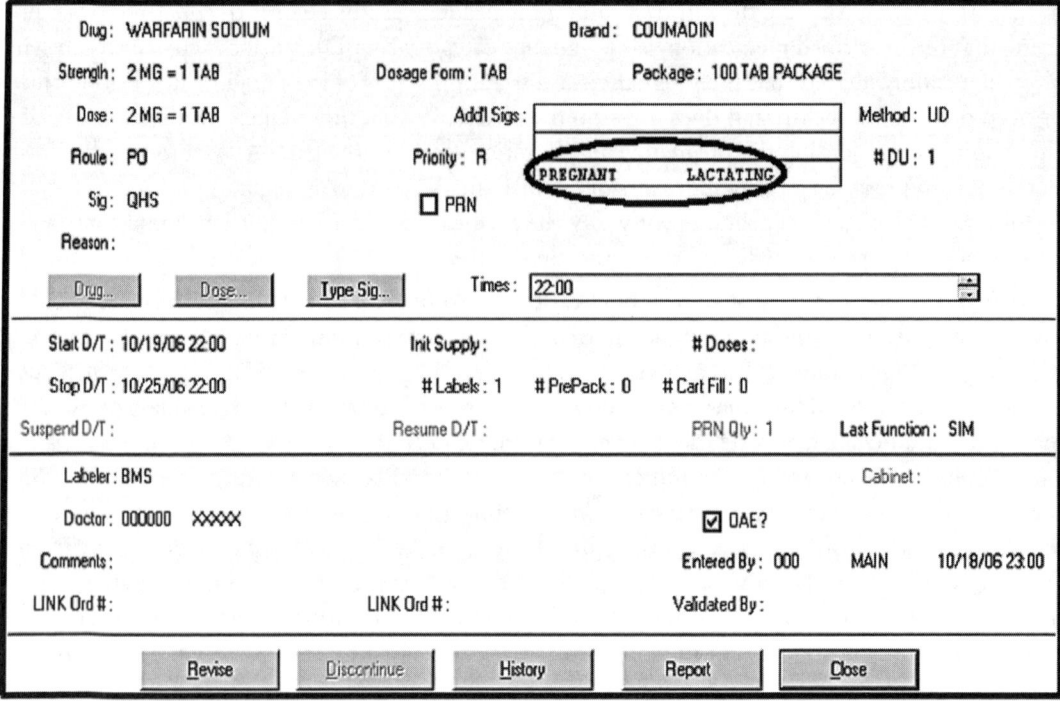

Figure 10.5. The Pregnancy and Lactation Status of the Patient Interfaces from the Directions Field of the CPOE System to the "Add'l Sigs" Field of the Pharmacy Application.

Conclusion

At KJMC, the pregnancy and lactation status of every female patient between the ages of 12 and 50 is completed during the initial assessment by the admitting nurse. The information that is obtained is readily available to the physician and nurse in the CPOE system, to the nurse in the MAK system, and to the pharmacist in the pharmacy application. All pregnancy category X or D medications that are part of the drug master file of the computer system are flagged to alert the physician and pharmacist that the pregnancy and lactation status of the patient must be documented prior to prescribing, verifying, and dispensing such medication. The pharmacist is ultimately responsible for approving a physician's order for a pregnancy category X or D drug in a pregnant or lactating patient.

Reference

1. Centers for Medicare and Medicaid Services (CMS). Specifications manual for national hospital quality measures, version 1.04. Washington, DC: Centers for Medicare and Medicaid Services, The Joint Commission on Accreditation of Healthcare Organizations (JCAHO); 2005.

Could Our Computer Help Us Comply with National Quality Standards?

David Merryfield

The Setting

Sentara Healthcare is an 1,800+ bed, 7-hospital, integrated healthcare system in southeastern Virginia and northeastern North Carolina. As one of the top-performing healthcare systems in the country, Sentara benchmarks against national quality indicators and was awarded the American Hospital Association Quest for Quality Award in 2004. Sentara provides pharmaceutical care via an innovative practice model, including deployed clinical pharmacists providing extensive, well-established clinical services in all patient care areas; the use of knowledge-based computer systems; and automated dispensing.

Sentara's pharmacy information system also provides an advanced clinical screening and alerting system. The goal of this system is to reduce preventable adverse drug events (ADEs) in Sentara hospitals by automatically screening medication orders for appropriateness at the time of order entry, monitoring drug therapy after the orders are initiated, and alerting the pharmacist when potential drug-related problems are identified. Medication orders are screened against laboratory results, patient demographics, and other data using logical rules, and the pharmacist is alerted when a potential opportunity is identified to improve the care of the patient. This use of information technology and automation allows the pharmacist to work more consistently and productively to intervene on the patient's behalf, and educate physicians and nursing staff. The pharmacy information management system, Sunrise Clinical Manager (Eclipsys Corporation), also allows the pharmacist to monitor a larger number of patients than could be handled through routine, manual screening of voluminous reports, or all patients' charts and labs. Alerts are primarily generated through the pharmacy information system, although printed reports and pagers are occasionally utilized as well.

Like other healthcare institutions, Sentara is publicly measured against quality standards for medication use from the Centers for Medicare and Medicaid Services (CMS), third-party payors, and accreditation and regulatory agencies. In several cases this assessment results in pay for performance; reimbursement rates are directly related to Sentara's performance against these national quality standards. Sentara was also an alpha testing site in 2003 for the Joint Commission™ ICU quality indicator development.

The Question

Representatives from the quality management, medical, and nursing departments came to pharmacy for help in achieving compliance with these indicators. In some cases the indicators were new (e.g.,

ICU core measures), but in some cases progress to date on achieving compliance with established indicators had been limited (e.g., heart failure medication use). Sentara's goal is not only to meet the standards, but also to be in the top 10% of hospitals nationally. So pharmacy was asked the following:

- "Can't pharmacists intervene to get the patients on the correct medications?"
- "Could our computer help us identify patients not on the correct medications?"

    The pharmacy determined that some of the medication use indicators listed below could be addressed through the use of the clinical screening and alerting system.
- AMI 1 (aspirin on arrival)—All acute myocardial infarction (AMI) patients without aspirin contraindications should receive aspirin within 24 hours before or after hospital arrival.
- AMI 2 (aspirin prescribed at discharge)—All AMI patients without aspirin contraindications should be prescribed aspirin at hospital discharge.
- AMI 3/HF 3 (ACEI or ARB for LVSD)—All AMI/heart failure (HF) patients with left ventricular systolic dysfunction (LVSD) and without angiotensin converting enzyme inhibitor (ACEI) and angiotensin receptor blocker (ARB) contraindications should be prescribed an ACEI or ARB at hospital discharge.

    For purposes of this measure, LVSD is defined as chart documentation of a left ventricular ejection fraction less than 40% or a narrative description of left ventricular systolic function consistent with moderate or severe systolic dysfunction.
- AMI 5 (beta-blocker prescribed at discharge)—All AMI patients without beta-blocker contraindications should be prescribed a beta-blocker at hospital discharge.
- AMI 6 (beta-blocker at arrival)—All AMI patients without beta-blocker contraindications should receive a beta-blocker within 24 hours after hospital arrival.
- Ventilator patients receiving care in the ICU should receive stress ulcer prophylaxis (SUP).
- Ventilator patients receiving care in the ICU should receive venous thromboembolism (VTE) prophylaxis.
- Critical care patients on vasopressors should receive corticosteroid support.
- All surgical cases >30 minutes should receive VTE prophylaxis.

The Answer

Sentara's pharmacy staff designed and the information technology department programmed an electronic screening and alerting system intended to identify those patients not receiving the appropriate medications. At the time this process was developed, the pharmacy information system did not have coded diagnoses, so it was necessary in some cases to develop markers for the situations in which the medications are indicated. These clinical screens include the following:

- Troponin >2 ng/mL as a marker for AMI, and then screening for patients not receiving aspirin, beta-blockade, or ACEI/ARB/hydralazine/nitrate (excluding patients with allergies to these agents)
- Beta naturetic peptide >700 pg/mL, carvedilol, and heart failure order sets/teaching materials as markers for heart failure, and then screening for patients not receiving ACEI/ARB/hydralazine-nitrate (excluding patients with allergies to these agents).

Pharmacist feedback soon confirmed that these were relatively weak markers for heart failure, so later a specific yes/no question was added to the electronic admission history database to indicate presence or absence of heart failure. This refinement of the marker improved identification of heart failure patients.

- Ventilator charges as a marker for ventilator patients, and then screening for SUP and VTE prophylaxis (including compression stockings using charges as a marker)
- Patients receiving vasopressors for >48 hours in critical care, then screening for the absence of a cortisol result or against serum cortisol levels <25 mcg/dL, with no corticosteroids/mineralocorticoids. Conversely, screening for patients with serum cortosol >25 mcg/dL, and receiving corticosteroids/mineralocorticoids, to consider whether they should be discontinued.
- Postoperative patients (via interface from the surgery information system) with a surgery duration greater than 30 minutes screened against the absence of VTE prophylaxis

Pharmacists are alerted by the computer system, either at the time of order entry or when relevant laboratory results are available, if the patient does not appear to be receiving appropriate therapy according to the logic of the screening process. The pharmacist then assesses the patient on whom an alert has been received, in the course of routine drug therapy monitoring and determines whether the medication is indicated or contraindicated. The pharmacist contacts the prescriber for new or revised orders, as appropriate.

Results

Pharmacist interventions have made a valuable contribution to improving medication use. Sentara's performance has achieved the goal of being in the top 10% nationally for aspirin and beta-blockade at discharge (100%). ACEI/ARB use has improved to 97%, and VTE and stress ulcer prophylaxis are consistently provided to critical care patients. Critical care pharmacists found the alerts helpful as reminders for corticosteroid use (although the literature recommending corticosteroids in patients on pressors has changed somewhat since the program began). The surgical VTE prophylaxis project is newer, but seems likely to have an impact.

The Future

Sentara is implementing computerized physician order management (CPOM) in January 2008. The integrated medical record will include coded diagnoses, which will improve the accuracy of these alerts and allow pharmacy to develop others. AMI versus the absence of statin use, VTE prophylaxis in patients with other high- and moderate-risk diagnoses, and other alerts are planned. The physician advisory group for the electronic medical record implementation has also determined that physicians will receive these alerts as CPOM begins. Pharmacists will then review physician overrides for appropriateness when verifying orders.

Conclusion

Use of a computerized screening and alerting system does help identify medications that are absent and improve the pharmacists' efficiency and effectiveness as they intervene to improve medication use. This system is a valuable part of an overall effort to achieve excellence in medication use.

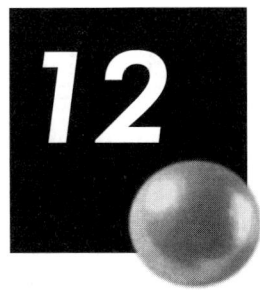

"If You Build It, Reports Will Come"

Susan J. Skledar
Kelly C. A. Ervin

Project Summary

This chapter describes a database solution for tracking formulary decisions at an academic medical center. With the increasing amounts of published literature, pharmacy departments and pharmacy & therapeutics (P&T) committees are challenged with updating and maintaining evidence-based formulary decisions. Medication formulary guidelines must be kept current, and this institution has created an electronic database solution for tracking formulary decisions that is able to generate reports on formulary reviews needing to be revised, numbers of reviews developed per year, and many other aspects of formulary and medication safety management.

Institution Description

The University of Pittsburgh Medical Center (UPMC) health system is a nonprofit, integrated healthcare delivery system and is comprised of a network of 19 hospitals and many other care sites across Western Pennsylvania and the world. Affiliated with the University of Pittsburgh Schools of the Health Sciences, it is the leading healthcare delivery system in Western Pennsylvania, consisting of a comprehensive network of community, specialty, and tertiary care hospitals; community-based programs; and a rapidly growing health insurance plan.[1] The UPMC Presbyterian hospital, the site of this intervention, is a 647-bed medical-surgical facility on the Oakland Campus of the health system. It is an academic teaching hospital serving patient populations such as those in transplantation, cardiothoracic surgery, internal medicine, geriatrics, critical care medicine and trauma, and cardiology. The pharmacy department offers services and clinical programs such as an investigational drug service, a poison and drug information center, a fully computerized unit-dose and intravenous admixture service, automated dispensing and robotic systems, anesthesiology/operating room satellite pharmacies, a decentralized pharmacy care model, an antibiotic management program, clinical faculty specialties (e.g., critical care, transplantation, surgery/trauma, neurovascular care, internal medicine, geriatrics, diabetes management, infectious diseases, drug information, ambulatory care), and a nationally recognized drug use and disease state management (DUDSM) program.[2]

DUDSM Program

Implemented in 1996, the DUDSM program was created as a medication-use policy, formulary management, and patient safety program. The goal of the program was to promote safe medication practices by using principles of evidence-based medicine to design clinical practice guidelines that optimize patient pharmacotherapy regimens, with all of this being done under the auspices of continuous quality improvement. Additional goals were to evaluate care processes and outcomes of identified disease states and evaluate the economic impact of drug therapies and their role in disease state management.

Originally known as a "target drug" or drug use evaluation program, the DUDSM program has, since 1996, greatly expanded its scope and has been responsible for design, implementation, and evaluation of nearly 300 guidelines (average of 30 per year) in the categories of patient safety, therapeutic interchange, disease state management, operational improvements, dose/route optimization, and off-label use of medications.[2,3] Faculty in the DUDSM program, along with additional clinical faculty, pharmacy residents, hospital-based clinical pharmacists, pharmacy technicians, and student pharmacists work collaboratively with physicians, nurses, and other members of the healthcare team to design these guidelines. Many of the guidelines have been published and have also served to set a medication safety and research agenda for the program.[3-10] Work has been done, for example, in the area of inpatient vaccination [4,8,10] and off-label use of medications.[3,9]

Background

One of the biggest challenges with sustaining a DUDSM program is to keep the content of the evidence-based guidelines current with the ever-growing quantity of published literature and changes in clinical practice. To address this challenge, the pharmacy DUDSM team at the UPMC Presbyterian Hospital developed a systematic process to review and update each guideline, through a periodic review of the underlying evidence base.[3,11,12] Another challenge is how to successfully implement the guidelines across the hospital, ensuring that physicians, nurses, pharmacists, and other members of the interdisciplinary healthcare team are able to access the guidelines and easily incorporate them into their everyday practice. The DUDSM guideline implementation process at UPMC includes the use of written, verbal, and electronic educational strategies. For example, formulary guidelines are implemented as standing orders, automatic interchanges, and through traditional mechanisms such as face-to-face discussions and phone calls with the medical staff. Prescribing compliance with the guidelines, drug utilization trends, and economic parameters such as drug cost per patient day and expense variance per fiscal year are monitored via the hospital's medical archive database and electronic health record. The internal threshold for compliance with the DUDSM guidelines is set at 85%, which has been achieved for the majority of guidelines in the program.

Although there are several challenges with maintaining a DUDSM program as noted above, the most critical is that the guidelines remain current and reflect the latest evidence in the literature. Studies have shown that barriers to successful implementation of clinical practice guidelines include lack of scientific robustness, outdated information, and the inability to understand and/or access the guidelines,[13,14] which reinforces the need to keep developed guidelines current. In its *Technical Assistance Bulletin on Drug Formularies*, the American Society of Health-System Pharmacists notes the need to keep formulary guidelines current by recommending that there should be a system for periodic revision and update of the formulary, usually annually.[15] Two of the Joint Commission™ medication management standards, MM.1.2.0, and MM.7.10., make recommendations regarding criteria for drug use and formularies.[16] The first states that medical staff members are to be involved in developing drug use criteria for medications available for dispensing, and also notes that these criteria are reviewed at least annually based on new efficacy and/or safety information. The latter recommends that processes for managing high-risk/high-alert medications are implemented. In the early years of the DUDSM program, several text-based documents, lists, and spreadsheets were created and maintained that outlined formulary guidelines approved and implementation dates each year. The internal need to keep the years of DUDSM evidence-based guidelines current, combined with ASHP and Joint Commission recommendations prompted creation of a system for formally tracking formulary decisions: **a formulary decision database**. This intervention is the topic of this safety-quality Pearl.

The Intervention

Staff in the DUDSM program designed an Access™ database (Microsoft Access, 2003. Microsoft Corporation) for this project. The decision to use an Access™ database allowed creation of customized reports, drop down menus, and easy functionality. The database was built to generate standard reports easily, consistently, and completely. Any new reports that are needed can be designed as well, as Access™ databases are very customizable. Key elements of the database included the following fields which were completed for each formulary decision/guideline at the facility: drug/disease state, guideline author, physician sponsor, type of guideline (e.g., therapeutic interchange, off-label use, patient safety, etc.), high-alert medication designation (based on the hospital's approved high-alert medication list), decision approval date, implementation strategy (e.g.,. automatic protocol, physician order set, restriction to prescriber service, etc.), implementation date, reference tool checklist (e.g., posting in on-line formulary, pharmacy department intranet Web page, teaching materials, physician electronic mail alert, etc.), date that followup is due back to the P&T committee, and dates of periodic updates. There is also a free-text box where other miscellaneous information can be entered, for example, a change of recommendation, or an action for a high-alert medication.

Figure 12.1 shows the entry page of the database. Navigation buttons allow five different actions: enter/edit initiative (guideline) data; choose a form; choose a report; access the p (shared) drive, which is the internal shared network drive containing full-text P&T committee/DUDSM teaching materials; and exit the database. This screen is accessed by anyone as they first enter the database to input new/updated guideline information, create a new form, or run a standard or custom report. Figure 12.2 shows the screen the user sees when he/she selects the Enter/Edit Initiative Data button on the entry page of the database. After each monthly formulary subcommittee (the "pre- P&T committee") meeting, an entry for each formulary guideline proposal is made into the database by a pharmacist on the DUDSM team. In the Enter/Edit Initiative Data screen, all fields are completed except for the P&T approval date, which is updated after the P&T committee formal decision is rendered. From Figure 12.2, fields completed include, for example, the author(s) name, the physician contact, initiative category, other interdisciplinary colleagues that have provided input into the guideline, committee approval dates, implementation strategies, and implementation dates. There is also a free-text field that can be used to update important information related to the formulary decision, for example, reasons for the topic being tabled or made nonformulary, or followup actions suggested. Guidelines that are tabled, or formulary requests that are denied,, are also entered into the database. Additionally in the database, on the Enter/Edit Initiative Data screen, there is also a field to indicate if a guideline is no longer active (e.g., drug removed from the market), which will remove it from any subsequent reports generated.

An automatic 1-year annual review date is attached to each entry, which will trigger a report that can be generated to display guidelines that need to be revised on an annual basis. To prepare in advance for these annual reviews, a report of Reviews [due] in 6 Months has also been created (see Figure 12.3). This report is generated by the DUDSM program director to help assign and prioritize writing projects for faculty, residents, and student pharmacists. For some of the formulary decisions made, the P&T committee requests that the topic come back to the committee in a timeframe shorter than 1 year, most often requested within 6 months, particularly in cases where data are limited, additional research on drug utilization is needed, cases of off-label medication use, or where coming therapeutic advances/literature are pending. The 6-month report tracks actions for the specific instances where the P&T committee votes that an update more frequently than the 1-year time-frame frame is needed. If the drug is indicated as "yes" on the 6-month report, then an update is due back to the P&T committee within 6 months of the formulary decision rendered (see Figure 12.3).

When the user selects the Choose a Report button, there are several standard reports that can be run. The standard reports are Annual Reviews Due, Reviews in 6 Months, Reviews by Category, and High-Alert Medications. To create additional, custom reports, for example, a list of approved/presented innovative off-label guidelines, the user can select Choose a Form to run a query and build the reports. For the aforementioned standard reports, each has a distinct purpose in maintaining the formulary system. The Annual Reviews Due and Reviews in 6 Months reports reveal information as to which guidelines have not been reviewed recently. As noted above, these reports are generated multiple times per year to set the agenda for pharmacy resident, student pharmacist, and faculty formulary writing projects. The annual report helps with yearly planning for writing projects, while the 6-month report is run at shorter intervals to help prioritize writing work. Pharmacy faculty in the DUDSM program are able to query these reports to create a worklist for literature updates as

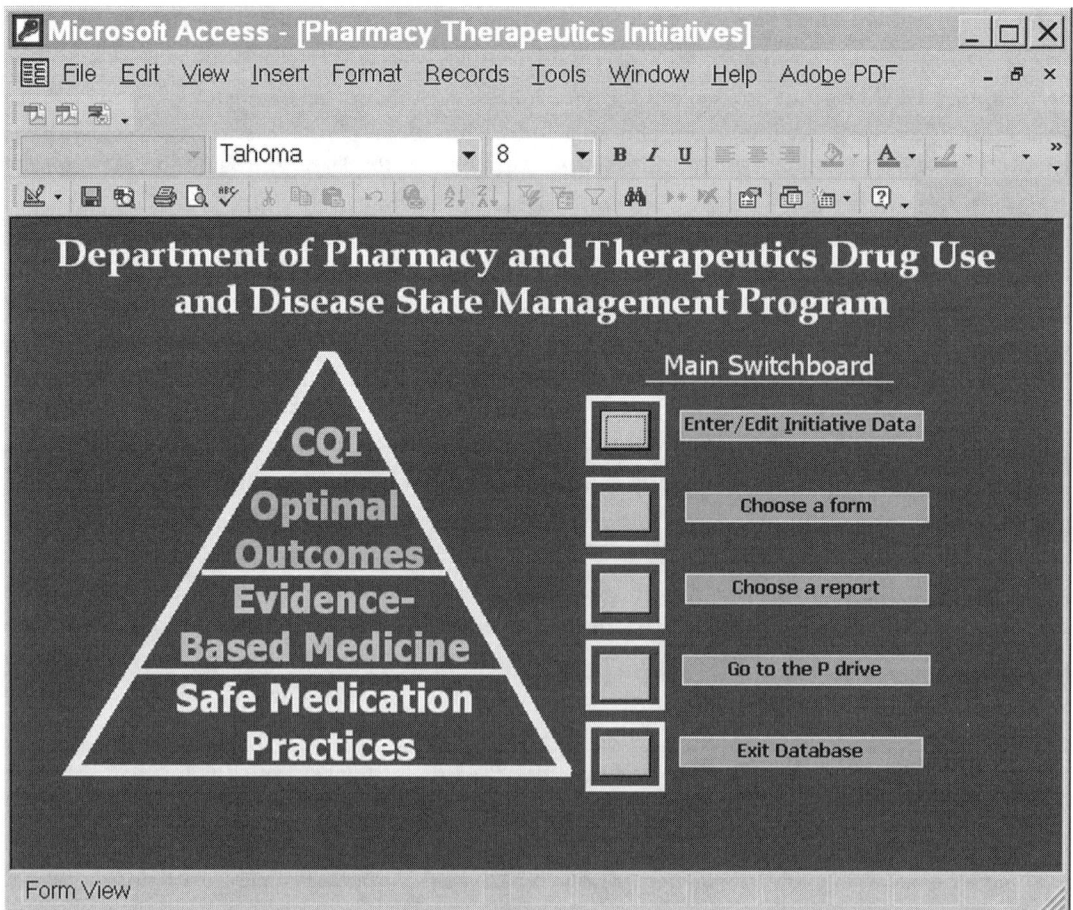

Figure 12.1. Entry Page of Formulary Decision Database.

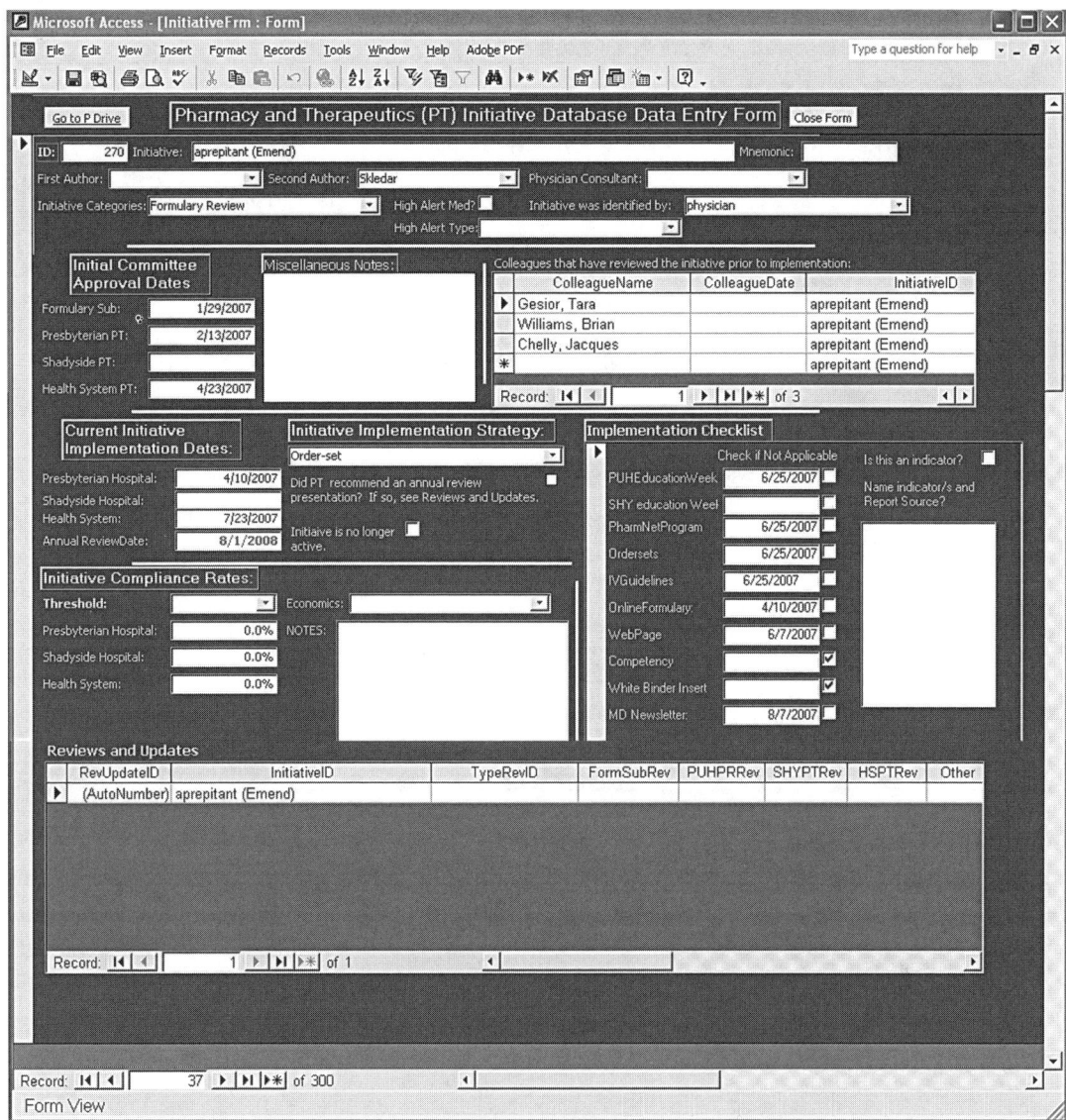

Figure 12.2. Screen for Entering/Editing an Initiative (Guideline) in the Database.

well. The Reviews by Category report is used by the DUDSM program director to create an annual summary of the productivity of the DUDSM program, for example, how many of each type of guideline was approved and implemented, and major categories of guidelines developed. This information is shared regularly with new pharmacists and faculty, the P&T committee, various quality committees in the institution, and for the departmental annual report. The High-Alert Category report was created to be an on-going chronicle of actions taken related to high-risk, high-alert medications such as anticoagulants and opioids.[17] Any of the standard or customized reports can be generated as an Access™ report or imported to a spreadsheet if needed. In the free-text section of the database on the Edit/Enter Initiative Data screen, the pharmacy manager of medication patient safety[18] enters high-alert actions (denoted as "haa" on the report) into the database. An example of such a high-alert action that would be logged into the database is creation of a preprinted order set for patient-controlled analgesia or prescribing service formulary restriction for factor concentrate

Reviews in 6 Months

PT Recommend	Annual Review Date	Initiative
Yes	1/1/2008	Levetiracetam (Keppra) IV and oral
Yes	1/1/2008	Ranolazine (Ranexa)
No	12/1/2007	Drotrecogin alfa (Xigris)
No	1/1/2008	Aprotinin guidelines
No	1/1/2008	Vitamin K guidelines

Figure 12.3. Report: Reviews Due in 6 Months.

products to ensure safety. Reports are run as needed, and are especially beneficial during Joint Commission or Department of Health inspections. During regulatory visits, pharmacy administrators are often asked to provide information and evidence that their hospital is taking action to ensure safety of high-alert medications; this report can be run at any time to provide such documentation. Figures 12.3 though 12.5 show samples of the reports above.

Conclusion

Since formulary guidelines are continually developed and implemented, the proactive P&T committee must keep the evidence review current, and a tracking system is essential to doing this successfully. Studies have shown that guidelines will be not successful if practitioners doubt their validity.[13,14] The formulary decision database has helped to achieve this goal of having the most current and best evidence translated into formulary decision-making and has not only improved the efficiency of the guideline update process, but has also allowed for report generation to categorize past and future actions.

Categories

Category	Disease Man/Patient Safety

Initiative

1. Surgical Prophylaxis Guidelines
2. Acute Insomnia Guidelines

Category	Disease Management

Initiative

1. Stress Ulcer Prophylaxis Guidelines
2. Aspiration Pneumonia
3. Heparin Induced Thrombocytopenia (HIT) Guidelines
4. Nosocomial Pneumonia
5. Community Acquired Pneumonia (CAP) Guidelines
6. ICU Paralytic Guidelines (NMBA)
7. Home Treatment of DVT with LMWH
8. Voriconazole Guidelines
9. Oncology Antiemetic Guidelines (5HT3)
10. Ulcer Disease Practice Guidelines
11. Contrast Nephropathy Prevention (RCN Prevention)
12. Post Operative Nausea Vomitting (PONV) Treatment Guidelines
13. Comfort Measures Order Set
14. Seizure Management Guidelines
15. Anemia Guidelines and Order Set
16. Gram Positive Treatment Algorithm
17. *Clostridium difficile*–Associated Disease (CDAD) Guidelines
18. Ventilator Associated Pneumonia
19. Telithromycin (Ketek)

Figure 12.4. Report: Reviews by Category.

High-Alert Report

High-Alert Med: Yes

Initiative	Category	Strategy	PUH Start	SHY Start	MiscNotes
3% Sodium Chloride Injection	Patient Safety				1) Only stocked and dispensed by pharmacy 2) 3/11/05 due to med event sent med safety alert to staff pharmacists 3) The pharmacy computer generated label has a note on the label itself—'Infuse via Central Line' for eMAR PPID units this would show up on the MAR and in EMTEK and ICU.
Adrenergic Agonist	Patient Safety	Operational Change	1/1/1992		haa: 1. Implemented standard infusion list in 1990 and revised yearly, including safety update in 3/06 2. Use premix solutions where available 3. Dose range checks in EMTEK 4. PharmNet drip complexes built for RPH order entry (12/01)
Bivalirudin Monograph/ Practice Guidelines	Patient Safety	Restrict to MD Service—COAG	10/1/2001	10/15/2001	haa: 1) Expanded use approved for HIT management (see HIT guidelines): 6/04

Figure 12.5. Report: High-Alert Medications (list adapted from reference 17).

References

1. About UPMC. Available at: http://www.upmc.com/home.htm. Accessed August 18, 2007.

2. Skledar SJ, Hess MM. Implementation of a drug-use and disease-state management program. *Am J Health Syst Pharm.* 2000;57(suppl 4):S23-S29.

3. Ansani N, Sirio C, Smitherman T, et al. Designing a strategy to promote safe, innovative off-label use of medications. *Am J Med Qual.* 2006;21:255-261.

4. Skledar SJ, Hess MM, Ervin KA, et al. Designing a hospital-based pneumococcal vaccination program. *Am J Health Syst Pharm.* 2003;60:1471-1476.

5. Tortorici MA, Skledar S, Barnes B, et al. Promoting the safe use of intravenous colchicine. *Am J Health Syst Pharm.* 2004;61:2496, 2501.

6. Sheth HS, Verrico MM, Skledar SJ, et al. Promethazine adverse events after implementation of a medication shortage interchange. *Ann Pharmacother.* 2005;39:255-261. Epub 2005 Jan 11.

7. Culley CM, Bernardo JF, Gross PR, et al. Implementing a standardized safety procedure for continuous renal replacement therapy solutions. *Am J Health Syst Pharm.* 2006;63:756-763.

8. Sokos DR, Skledar SJ, Ervin KA, et al. Designing and implementing a hospital-based vaccine standing orders program. *Am J Health Syst Pharm.* 2007;64:1096-1102.

9. Juang P, Skledar SJ, Zgheib NK, et al. Clinical outcomes of intravenous immune globulin in severe clostridium difficile-associated diarrhea. *Am J Infect Control.* 2007;35:131-137.

10. Middleton DB, Fox DE, Nowalk MP, et al. Overcoming barriers to establishing an inpatient vaccination program for pneumococcus using standing orders. *Infect Control Hosp Epidemiol.* 2005;26:874-881.

11. Ansani NT, Fedutes-Henderson BA, Skledar SJ, et al. Practical approach to grading evidence for formulary recommendations. *Am J Health Syst Pharm.* 2005;62:1498-1501.

12. Corman SL, Skledar SJ, Culley CM. Evaluation of conflicting literature and application to formulary decisions. *Am J Health Syst Pharm.* 2007;64:182-185.

13. Cabana MD, Rand CS, Powe NR, et al. Why don't physicians follow clinical practice guidelines? A framework for improvement. *JAMA.* 1999;282:1458-1465.

14. Ellrodt G, Cook DJ, Lee J, et al. Evidence-based disease management. *JAMA.* 1997;278;1687-1692.

15. American Society of Hospital Pharmacists. ASHP technical assistance bulletin on drug formularies. *Am J Hosp Pharm.* 1991;48:791-793.

16. The Joint Commission. *2006 Comprehensive Accreditation Manual for Hospitals: The Official Handbook* (CAMH). Oakbrook Terrace, IL: The Joint Commission; 2006.

17. ISMP's List of High-Alert Medications. Available at: http://www.ismp.org/Tools/highalert-medications.pdf. Accessed August 18, 2007.

18. Kowiatek JG, Weber RJ, Skledar SJ, et al. Medication safety manager in an academic medical center. *Am J Health Syst Pharm.* 2004;61:58-64.

Quality, Near and Far

John M. Petrich

Introduction

Investigators at an academic medical center may prefer to store and dispense their own ambulatory study medications instead of using the institution's pharmacy. While storage and dispensing by investigators may prove to be more convenient or less costly, it does not necessarily conform to the Joint Commission™ standards and introduces the risk of errors and deficiencies. Accordingly, a rigorous quality review of nonpharmacy investigational drug handling is essential.

At Cleveland Clinic the quality review program is a Department of Pharmacy initiative designed to address specific Joint Commission medication management standards. Because the pharmacy staff believed physician investigators and research coordinators might need assistance meeting the Joint Commission standards related to pharmacy practice, the formalization of a quality review program began in 2001. The quality review program is intended to monitor compliance with Joint Commission standards associated with drug handling, especially relating to investigator controlled research medications. Specifically, the Investigational Drug Service (IDS) performs quarterly reviews of the drug storage, study documentation, and regulatory compliance of all drugs under the institution's umbrella. Joint Commission has verbalized its support for Cleveland Clinic's quality review program as a means to deal with the institution's unique makeup, broad scope, and vast landscape.

A quality review program within a hospital pharmacy can enhance the integrity of clinical trials at several levels. This chapter defines the role of the Cleveland Clinic's quality review program, identifies key components of compliance with applicable Joint Commission standards, and describes the impact of Cleveland Clinic's quality review program over time. The mechanism by which the program was implemented and the tools used to complete the tasks are also described.

Quality Measurement at Cleveland Clinic

Cleveland Clinic has approximately 1,000 inpatient beds. In 2001 this institution had more than 52,000 hospital admissions and 2.5 million outpatient visits, with patients from every state and more than 90 countries.[1] Also in 2001 there were more than 700 institutional review board (IRB) approved studies among 90 specialties and subspecialties at Cleveland Clinic. Investigators stored and dispensed the drugs for about one-third of the outpatient studies and the pharmacy controlled the drugs for the remainder. The pharmacy stored and dispensed investigational drugs for all inpatient studies.

Department policy states that the IDS is responsible for the quality of all study drug supplies regardless of who stores and dispenses the medication and where these functions are performed. The IDS is comprised of five full-time professionals: the service coordinator, a pharmacist, and three research technicians. IDS staff members work closely with many investigators and research coordinators, staff pharmacists, technicians, and other support staff. In addition to storage, dispensing, and quality review, the IDS has the ability to perform drug accountability, inventory management, randomization and blinding services, audit preparedness, and disseminate drug information for industry-sponsored, government-sponsored, physician-initiated, and cooperative group studies within the institution.

Predictably, oversight of pharmacy controlled study drugs is relatively simple and quality standards are met rather easily. However, the real focus of the quality review program is on study drug that the investigators store and dispense from remote locations.

A significant challenge at Cleveland Clinic is the assurance of quality across its vast network. There are several family health centers and clinics throughout suburban Cleveland that may conduct clinical research. The IDS must find a way to integrate all remote drug studies into the quality review program. The task confronting the IDS is to develop quality review processes that apply to the entire network, and to implement those processes in a meaningful way that can be measured.

The IDS has overcome many important challenges during the last decade. Enhanced communication between the IRB, investigators, and the pharmacy is an example of one such triumph. IDS successfully lobbied for the inclusion of a line item within the new electronic IRB application that was recently launched at Cleveland Clinic. A line on the application now requires investigators to declare their intention regarding drug handling, and this information is automatically communicated to the pharmacy for every IRB-approved study. The IDS has complete confidence that all study drugs are being reviewed for quality, due to the revised IRB application and the resultant required communication. Before this change, several studies would slip through the cracks and not be evaluated in the quality review process. The opportunity to be notified at the level of the IRB application essentially enables the IDS to guide an investigator into making the best choice for the handling of his or her study drug. Any investigator who intends to manage the drugs independent from the pharmacy is asked to consider a set of criteria (Figure 13.1) to ensure that they have the proper resources to safely and effectively carry out such management. The IDS requires investigators to relinquish control of the study drugs when the product requires sterile preparation or for any inpatient study.

The Quality Review Worksheet

Quality measurement requires an instrument or a tool. The quality measurement tool of the Cleveland Clinic IDS is the Quality Review Worksheet (Figure 13.2). Elements of the Quality Review

---

Criteria for Drug Control

- Pharmacy control of study drug
  - inpatient studies
  - sterile preparation, sterile technique
  - blinding
  - repackaging, labeling
  - space
  - time and resources

- Investigator control with remote, periodic pharmacy monitoring
  - outpatient studies
  - oral drug packaged and labeled for dispensing
  - convenience factor
  - no need for the resources listed in pharmacy criteria

Figure 13.1. Criteria for Drug Control.

Worksheet are derived from study drug storage and accountability accreditation standards.

IDS staff members use the Quality Review Worksheet to conduct quarterly audits of study drug storage, accountability, and regulatory documentation. The Quality Review Worksheet starts with study-specific demographic data and then covers three sections: investigational medication storage, investigational medication refrigerators, and investigational records. IDS staff answer a series of questions related to each section; acceptable answers are "yes," "no," or "N/A."

The first section pertains to investigational medication storage. Temperature in the medication storage area should be documented. Historically, the lack of this documentation has been a frequent deficiency, especially for drugs that should be stored at room temperature. Medications

Quality Review Worksheet

The Cleveland Clinic Foundation Department of Pharmacy
Investigational Drug Inspection

Location:_____Study Title_____
Date_____
Activity # _____   Cost Center # _____

For new studies initiated after November 1, 2002

Investigational Medication Storage	YES	NO	N/A
1. Room temperature documented in medication storage area	___	___	___
2. Investigational Medications storage area secured with limited access.	___	___	___
3. Investigational Medications requiring special conditions (i.e., room temp., refrigeration, protected from light, etc. are properly stored	___	___	___
4. Investigational medications are properly labeled for investigational use @ and are separate from other noninvestigational drugs.	___	___	___
5. Investigational medications are in date.	___	___	___
6. Returns and expired investigational medications identified and separate from active inventory.	___	___	___

Investigational Medication Refrigerators	YES	NO	N/A
1. Refrigerator is stored in a secure area with limited access.	___	___	___
2. Refrigerator is clean and does not contain excessive frost.	___	___	___
3. Operating at proper temperature (36–46°F; 2–8°C).	___	___	___
4. A Temperature log is being kept.	___	___	___
5. Investigational medications under refrigeration are properly labeled and separate from noninvestigational drugs.	___	___	___
6. Refrigerator does not contain food or other nondrug items.	___	___	___
7. Investigational medications are in date.	___	___	___
8. Returns kept under refrigeration are identified and stored separate.	___	___	___

Investigational Records	YES	NO	N/A
1. A current copy of protocol available and kept in a secure area.	___	___	___
2. A current IRB letter of approval is on file.	___	___	___
3. IRB Number	___	___	___
4. The IRB annual progress report for renewal or final report of completion is due on or before _____ (date).			
5. Names of investigator, coordinator and sponsor are available: Principal Investigator:_____ Study coordinator:_____	___	___	___
6. Pertinent information on study medication available for patient.	___	___	___
7. Consent forms are being obtained on every subject prior to enrolling the subject into the study and are kept in a secure area.	___	___	___
8. Documentation is being completed/signed by authorized personnel	___	___	___
9. Records of shipment from suppliers are kept.	___	___	___
10. Dispensing log is being kept and coincides with the current inventory	___	___	___
11. Destruction is being done per FDA regulations and per sponsors wishes	___	___	___

Investigator signature _____ Date _____
Investigational Drug Service   pager 21755

Figure 13.2. Quality Review Worksheet.

must be stored in a secured area with limited access and should be in date. During the quarterly review program's infancy, expired medications were often found in medication storage areas. Returns and expired investigational medications should be identified and separated from active inventory. Study drugs should not be mixed in with samples or any other U.S. Food and Drug Administration (FDA) approved drugs.

Notable in section two of the Quality Review Worksheet, medication refrigerators should be in a secure area with limited access. They should operate at the proper temperature and be free of frost buildup. Temperature in these refrigerators should be monitored and a backup power supply should be available. Study drugs should be in date, identified, and stored separately from insulin, food, or pathology specimens.

The third section deals with regulatory documentation and accountability. A copy of the current protocol should be available and kept in a secure area. A current IRB approval letter should be on file. Pertinent information on the study medication should be available for patients. IDS staff members check to see that informed consent forms are being completed on every subject prior to enrollment, and that authorized personnel perform the informed consent documentation. They also check to see that records of shipments of study drugs from suppliers are kept, dispensing logs are being kept and coincide with inventory, and that destruction is done according to regulations and the study sponsor's wishes.

A "no" response on any category in the Quality Review Worksheet requires action. IDS staff members advise the study coordinator about deficiencies that require corrective action and ensure timely followup, typically within 1 to 2 weeks.

Additional services are provided on an "as needed" basis. For example, IDS may provide open text labels for products that may not meet labeling standards. Open text labels are a free-format label that allow the investigators to augment information to the patient and the healthcare team. Information that should be found on the label includes patient specific data, identity, strength, dose, quantity, and directions for administration of the investigational agent. The label should also include storage requirements for the medication, expiration dating, manufacturer information, and lot numbers. Lastly, the contact information of the investigator should be included in the labeling along with a clear statement that the medication is an investigational drug. This way, if a patient is admitted to a different healthcare facility, the attending physician can easily obtain information about the investigational drug. These elements meet the policy for investigational drug labeling at Cleveland Clinic.

IDS may provide access to thermometers and temperature graphs to chart drug storage conditions. IDS may also assist with drug destruction or provide necessary forms for documentation of destruction, transfer of product, or notes to file.

Findings

In 2001 the IDS set out to measure the impact of its newly created quality review program using the Quality Review Worksheet. The goals of the review are below:

- Measure the impact of the IDS quality review program on various elements found on the Quality Review Worksheet when drug is stored and dispensed outside of the pharmacy
- Prevent medication-related complications that would result from deficiencies found on the Quality Review Worksheet

The design of the small pilot project was relatively simple. The tool for the quality measurements was the Quality Review Worksheet. A finding of "no" on the worksheet requires corrective action and was referred to as a deficiency. After a round of quarterly reviews, the numbers of queries answered "no" on the worksheets were tallied. A year later, the process was repeated, and the results compared to the previous measurements.

Since the quality review program was absent at Cleveland Clinic prior to 2001, IDS believed that the impact of the program would be best illustrated by assessing its effectiveness just after implementation. Specifically, the level of deficiencies on the first inspection in 2001 was unacceptably high; however, since that time, the level of deficiencies has trended downward to a sustained negligible level. Therefore, the time point that best describes the IDS impact is at the beginning, during the inception of the program.

Figure 13.3 highlights the results of the pilot project. In the second quarter of 2001, IDS staff members counted 156 deficiencies among 174 worksheets. In the second quarter of 2002, IDS counted 57 deficiencies among 190 worksheets. Despite the increase in studies over the chosen timeframe, there was a dramatic decrease in the number of deficiencies recorded on the worksheets. This positive trend marks improvement in patient safety, investigator awareness, and accreditation compliance. IDS believes the decline in deficiencies is due, at least in part, to the educational component of the inspections. Over time, investigators and coordinators became familiar with the quality review checklist, and, therefore, became educated in the associated standards it contained.

To demonstrate that the quality improvement could be sustained over time, IDS staff members performed the measurements again in 2003 (Figure 13.4). Again, despite the increasing number of studies, the number of deficiencies continued to decline. Continuous quality improvement was

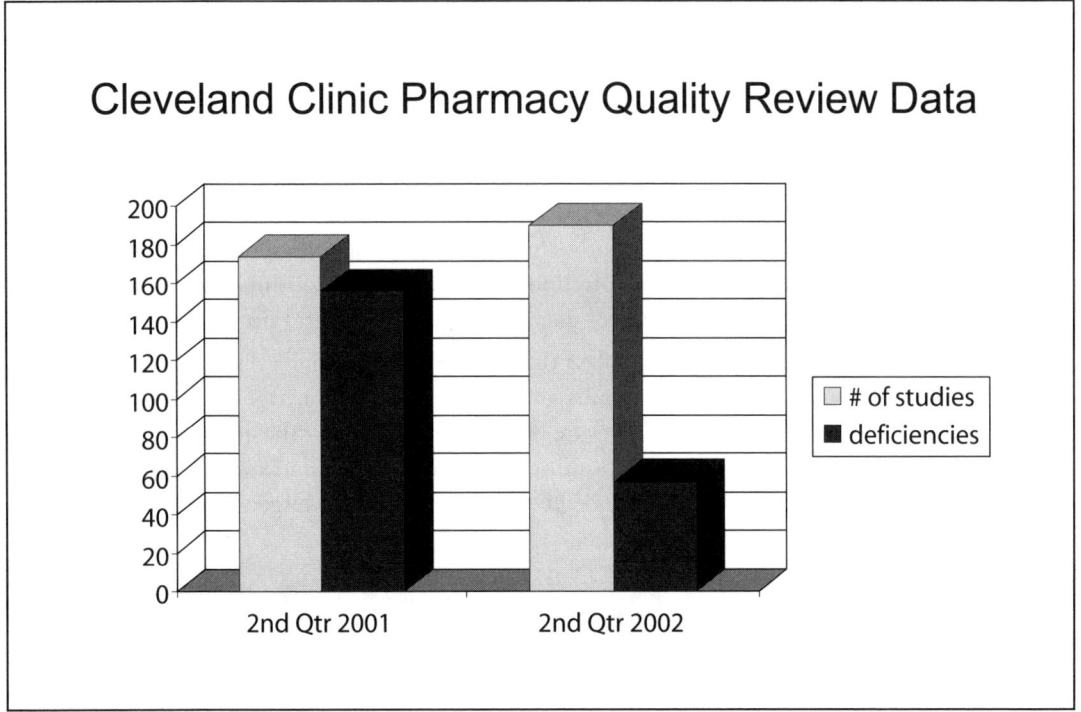

Figure 13.3. Quality Review Data, 2001–2002.

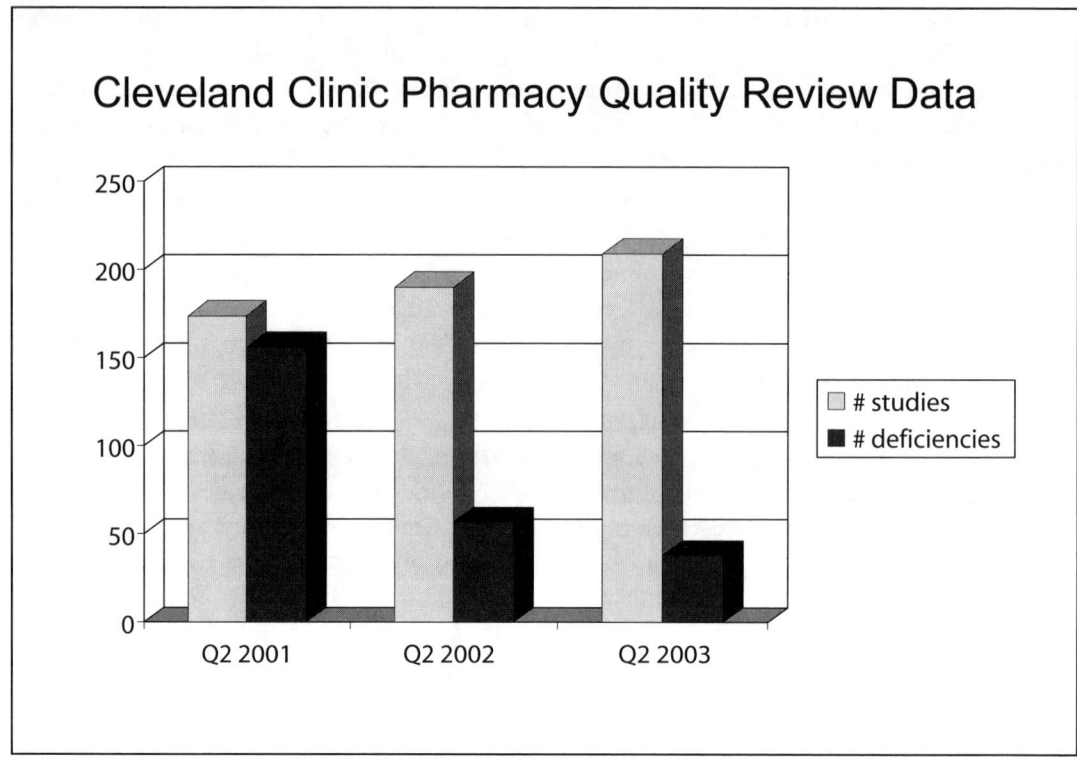

Figure 13.4. Quality Review Data, 2001–2003.

demonstrated as a decline in deficiencies among a rising number of worksheets for 2 consecutive years. The number one deficiency for all 3 years, "room temperature not documented," fell from 79% in 2001 to 14% in 2003.

Conclusion

The trend showing a decrease in deficiencies despite the increasing number of studies provides some evidence of the positive impact and professional value of the IDS upon the healthcare delivery system at Cleveland Clinic. Perhaps most importantly, these data may imply the power of education conveyed to investigators and coordinators involved in clinical research. Continuous improvement was demonstrated through 3 consecutive years of data showing a meaningful decrease in deficiencies.

The Joint Commission estimates that less than 5% of organizations do not comply with its standards. Most of those standards focus on patient safety and medication systems. Researchers handling investigational drugs may not be aware of these standards, but the quality review program at Cleveland Clinic indicates that quality monitoring is a meaningful endeavor. Although levels of errors and deficiencies are now very low, it is expected that continued diligence will be necessary to maintain the current level of quality.

Reference

1. Cleveland Clinic Intranet. Available at: http://www.clevelandclinic.org/. Accessed June 2002.

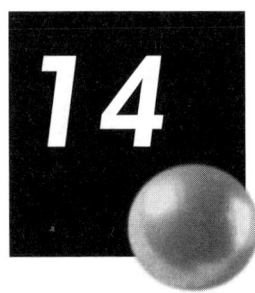

14

The www of Adverse Drug Reaction Reporting

Todd Lemke

No, this Pearl is not about a worldwide wrestling league developed to decide who is responsible for the lengthy documentation required for adverse drug reactions. Nor is it about a new upstart "dot com" company out to bring in large profits before going belly up in the late 90s. This Pearl is about a rural Minnesota hospital and the staff's desire to create a better way to report, store, group, and analyze adverse drug reactions that occur within the Paynesville Area Health Care System.

Paynesville Area Health Care System and Its Pharmacy Department

The Paynesville Area Health Care System is anchored by a 25-bed, critical access hospital with seven satellite clinics and two long-term care facilities all located in central Minnesota. The healthcare system serves a 50-mile radius containing approximately 25,000 people and is governed by elected representatives from the 12 cities and townships within this radius. The hospital has approximately 650 admissions each year with the outpatient services of the hospital and clinics having 250,000 clinical interactions with patients each year.*

The health system's pharmacy department is responsible for both clinical and dispensing duties in the hospital, long-term care facilities, and clinics. Three pharmacists and three technicians provide 10 hours of on-site availability each day for the hospital, nursing homes, and clinic. Pharmacists share on-call coverage for night and weekends when the pharmacy is closed. The department utilizes a pharmacy computer system for both the hospital and long-term care facilities. In the hospital, the automated drug distribution system, Omnicell, is utilized for the majority of medications given in the medical/surgical unit, emergency department, and surgery suites. The long-term care residents receive medications from unit-dose packaging.

These automation and medication distribution efficiencies allow the pharmacists to be more clinically involved in patient care in the hospital, long-term care facilities, and clinic. Pharmacists provide medication therapy management in all areas of the healthcare system. In the hospital they are involved in the monitoring and adjustment of medications based on patient condition changes, laboratory values, and evidence-based clinical guidelines. Protocols are in place for a pharmacist to assist in the clinical management of many health conditions for hospitalized patients. Long-term

---

*Admissions data were gathered from hospital and clinic patient census data provided by the Paynesville Area Health Care System business office.

care residents receive similar pharmacy clinical services with pharmacists being responsible for diabetes and anticoagulation management. The clinic is staffed 7 hours each day by a pharmacist that provides diabetes education, diabetes medication management, anticoagulation services, and medication therapy management.

The Dilemma

In 2003 the pharmacy director found that the methods of reporting actual medication errors and adverse drug reactions in the healthcare facility did not track and evaluate the reports. *Medication errors* are defined in the institution as errors involved in the ordering, transcribing, dispensing, and administration of medications. Medication errors include both errors that reach the patient and those that are caught before the medication reached or didn't reach the patient. *Adverse drug reactions* are defined as unexpected or dangerous reactions to a medication that changes the level of care being given to a patient. These adverse drug reactions could occur in the outpatient, inpatient, or long-term care setting. Each area, hospital, and long-term care and clinic, utilized different methods—some verbal and some written—for recording errors and adverse reactions. Reported medication errors and adverse drug reactions were in some instances handled by disciplinary action for the employee involved and in other instances were just filed in a folder. Consequently, there were few errors and adverse drug reactions reported. In total there were only three medication errors each month in the facility and no adverse drug reactions reported in the 4-year period prior to 2003. Compared with other facilities of similar size, there was either under reporting or a near perfect execution of patient care in the facility.

Pathway to the Solution

The pharmacy director brought the issue forward to the quality improvement committee, and a task force was formed to solve the problem. The task force included representatives from the pharmacy, nursing, quality improvement, staff education, medical records, and technology departments. The task force was charged with identifying one system for the entire facility that could be utilized for gathering medication errors and adverse drug reaction reports.

The task force identified three key issues that were possibly reducing the number of reports being submitted. One issue was that errors were treated as a punitive event. A nurse that had committed multiple errors was verbally reprimanded and, consequently, other errors in the facility went unreported. Unreported errors can lead to further errors, as many times a system or process is implicated in errors, instead of one individual's mistake. A second issue was the time and process involved in reporting the error or adverse reaction. Current processes required that the error or adverse reaction report be filled out by the person involved with the error, that the initial report be written in blue ink, and that all staff involved provide signatures. Error reporting was often put off and then sometimes forgotten. Another issue was that reports did not go to one central location but to individual department managers who might each deal with the report differently.

After much investigation, the task force decided the medication error and adverse reaction reporting system needed to have the following traits:

1. It should be easy to access.
2. The reporting tool should be short and simple to understand.
3. The reporting should be anonymous.

4. A climate of nonpunitive reporting should be developed.

5. The reports should go to one central location.

6. All staff should be trained on the reporting system.

7. When errors and reactions occurred, procedures and processes should be reviewed to see if the incident could be avoided next time.

8. The tool would not be paper-based.

The task force took the traits desired for the reporting system and began investigating what currently available reporting products would fit the needs of the facility, as resources were not available to create a system from scratch. After some research on the Web and at professional meetings such as the American Society of Health-Systems Pharmacists Midyear Clinical Meeting, two products were chosen for final review. The reporting products from Healthprolink (www.healthprolink.com) and Saferating (www.saferating.com) were evaluated both by online review and live Web demonstrations with each company. Both products met the needs of the pharmacy department but the other members of the task force felt that the Saferating product provided a more nurse-friendly product. In the end Saferating was chosen as the vendor to provide the medication error and adverse drug reaction reporting systems.

Implementing Saferating.com

The Saferating reporting tool is a Web-based reporting system that allows users to either utilize premade reporting templates or develop reporting tools from scratch. The site-specific reports are accessed through a secure Web site for incident report entry. The company is able to restrict access to the reporting tool to make it secure to an individual facility. Access to reports, once they are submitted, is through a password-protected secure server. Accessing this server, pharmacists, nursing directors, quality assurance staff, or other authorized individuals are able to create reports to look at individual entries or look for trends from groupings of entries.

The pharmacy department was charged with the task of developing the tools that individuals would use to report medication errors or adverse reactions. Using templates developed by Saferating, the pharmacy department individualized the form to meet some institution-specific needs. The reporting needed to record the location of the medication error or adverse drug reaction within the healthcare system (hospital, clinic, specialty services, long-term care facility) and break down into categories that allowed grouping of errors and adverse reactions to look for patterns. Once these specifics were decided, the Saferating staff provided the individualized Web page that would gather the data. Medication errors or adverse drug reactions are then entered through a link to a secure Web site. The link is available as a short cut on each staff member's computer desktop. Figures 14.1 through 14.5 demonstrate the Web site for the adverse reaction reporting tool.

The staff education department provided training to nursing, pharmacy and clinic staff that would be using the reporting system. The training involved all aspects of the system from utilizing Web pages for entering information to the correct way of entering a medication error or adverse drug reaction. The change to a nonpunitive culture was also stressed during training to encourage entry of not only errors, but also errors that were caught before they could cause harm. These types of errors were categorized as *near misses*. One interesting aspect of the education process was that many staff needed beginner level training in computer utilization. After training was rolled out in all departments, the Saferating product was put into effect.

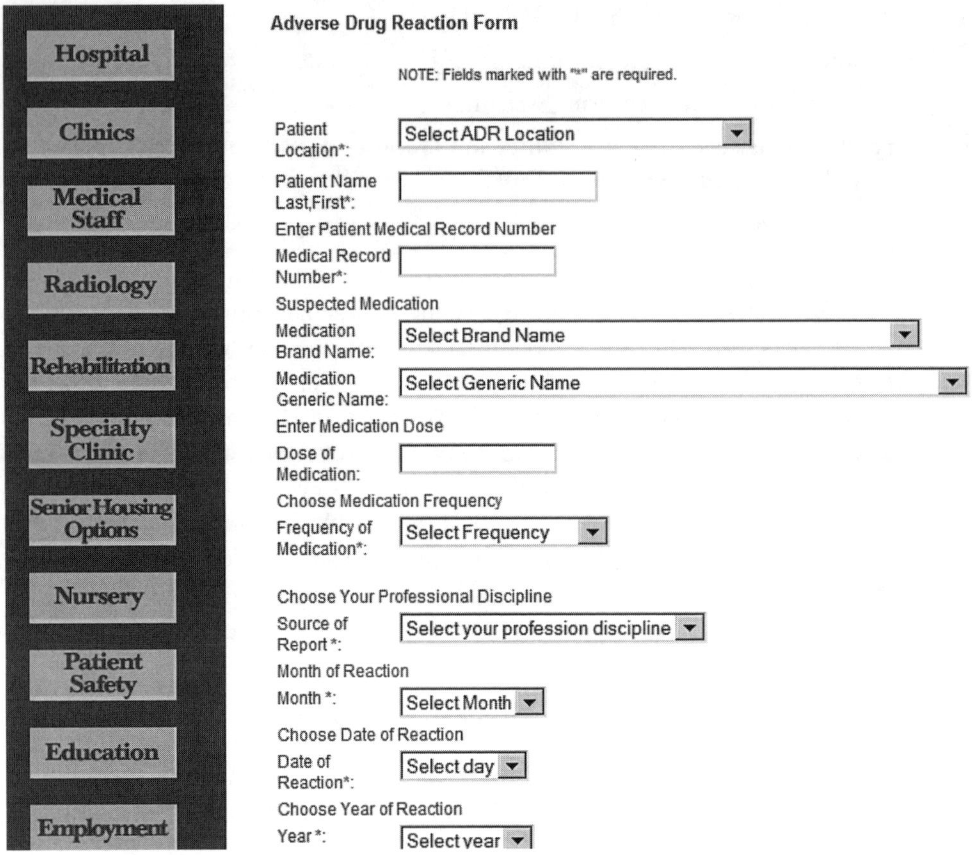

Figure 14.1. Screen opens directly from a nurse or pharmacist's desktop through the use of a quick link. The Web page includes drop-down boxes that can be utilized by the staff member to further define and describe the adverse drug reaction.

The reporting system was set up to send an email that an error or adverse drug reaction had occurred to the director of pharmacy. The pharmacy director would then review the report and forward it to the nursing director of the specific area that the error occurred in or investigate the adverse drug reaction further if needed. Monthly summaries of the reported errors and adverse reactions generated from the database are reviewed and presented to the pharmacy and therapeutics (P&T) committee. Quarterly, the quality improvement committee reviews trends in error and adverse drug reactions. When trends are found indicating potential errors and reactions could be prevented, the committee works with the involved departments to create a process change. The change is then monitored to see if medication errors or adverse drug reactions are decreased because of the change.

Analysis of the Reporting System

The pharmacy department director's review of the reporting system after 3 months of use already showed increased utilization over the previous reporting method. An average of 70 errors or near misses and three adverse drug reactions were reported each month. Staff members were rewarded with pizza for the way the process was being embraced. After 6 months certain adverse event/medication error reporting trends were seen, and processes, such as medication pass methods and standing order sets, were reviewed to find the point at which similar errors were occurring. In instances

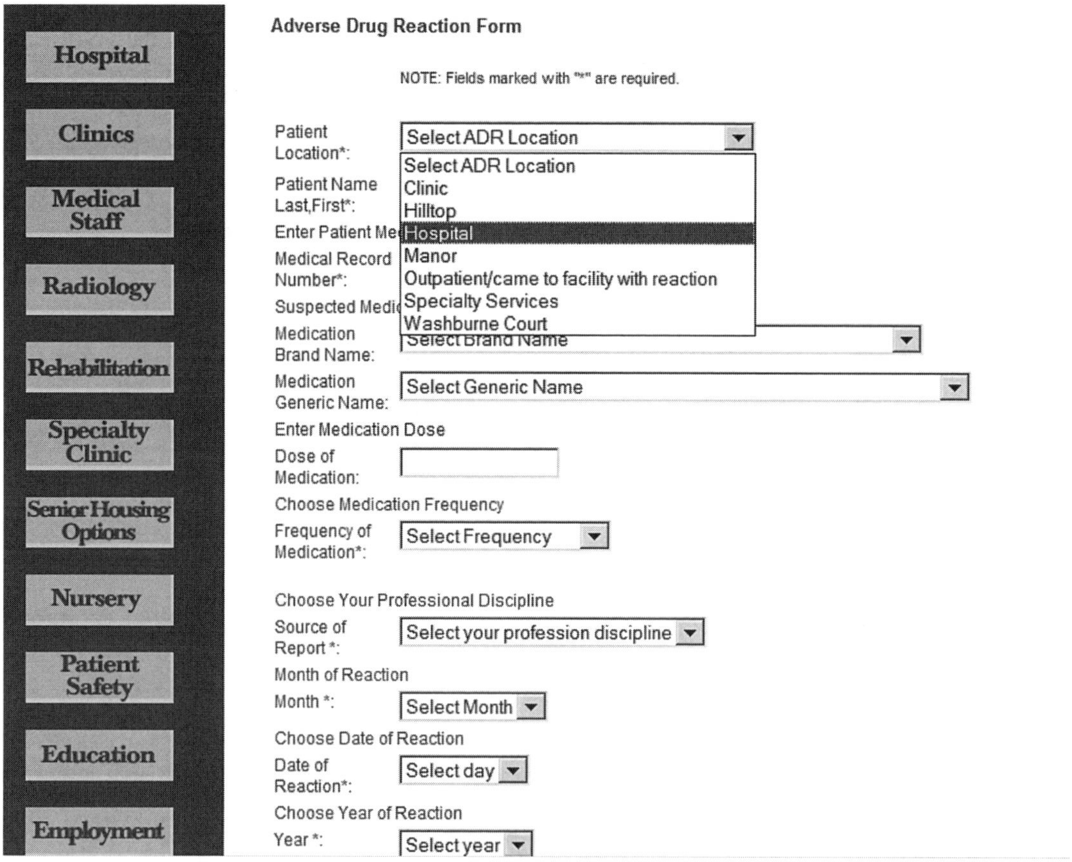

Figure 14.2. Drop-down boxes in this example allow the staff member entering the report to select the location of the reaction.

where similar errors occurred, orders sets were made clear or staff members were trained to change the behaviors that were creating the risk of an error occurrence.

For example, data from the new reporting system revealed a preventable adverse drug reaction that occurred in different patients three times in a 3-month period when the nursing department contacted on-call physicians after pharmacy hours. Specifically, the on-call physician ordered a second long-acting pain medication before the first long-acting analgesic achieved its therapeutic effect. As a result, the patient experienced increased sedation and decreased respiration rates. Utilizing the information obtained from the reporting system, the pharmacy and nursing departments made a change in hospital processes. Now, nurses must review patients' current medication profiles with the on-call physician (who may be unfamiliar with a patient's current medications) whenever a pharmacist is unavailable for prospective medication review.

In another example, review of data from the new reporting system revealed a medication error trend. There were several instances where incorrect doses had been administered. In each of these cases, the order had been for two tablets, but only one had been administered. Utilizing the data from the reporting system, the pharmacy department modified the medication administration record and placed an alert on the automated medication distribution system, Omnicell, to remind nursing staff when the dose was two or more tablets. The incidence of these types of errors decreased after the changes were implemented. Reported "incorrect dose given" instances went from 20 events each month to three events monthly when the data was reviewed at 6 months after intervention.

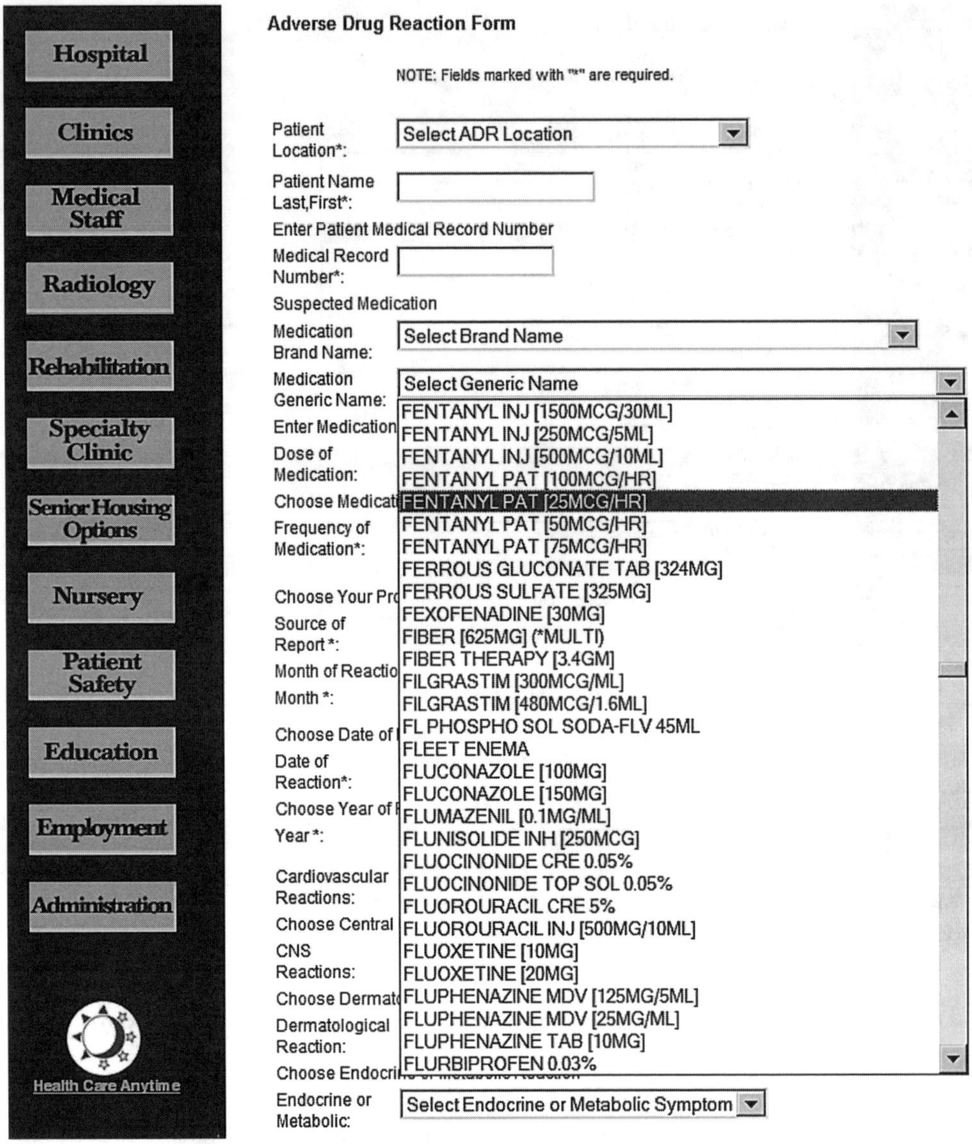

Figure 14.3. The facility's formulary is linked to the Web page with both generic and brand name designations for medications to allow for ease of use for nursing and other nonpharmacy staff.

Summary

After nearly 3 years of utilization of the Saferating adverse drug reaction and medication error reporting system, the pharmacy and nursing departments are still finding good use of the system. With over 1,000 reported medication errors (both errors occurring and near misses) and adverse drug reactions, the ability to look at trends in errors and adverse drug reactions has proven incredibly helpful in improving the patient care process and medication delivery system within the healthcare system. Further, use of the Saferating system has helped the health system be in compliance with a regulation for critical access hospitals, C-0277 485.635(a)(3)(v): *Procedures for reporting adverse drug reactions and errors in the administration of drugs.*

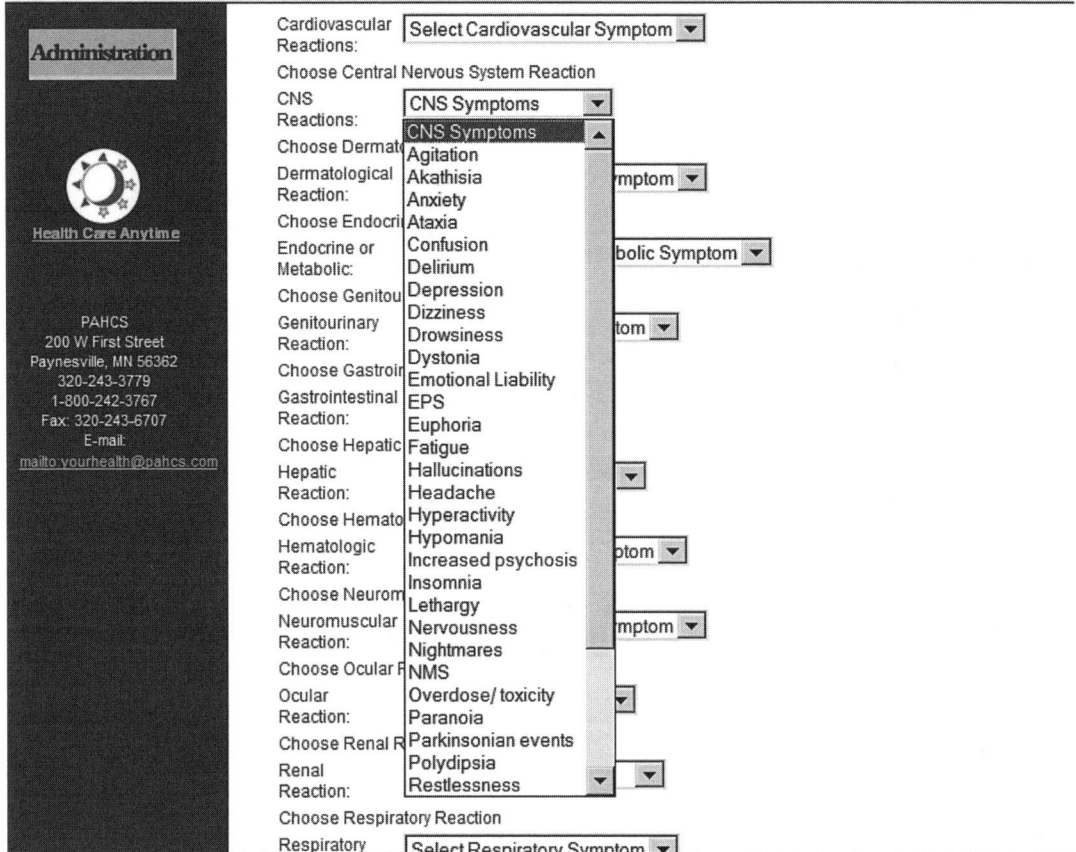

Figure 14.4. Specific symptoms of the reaction are recorded utilizing drop-down boxes by body system.

The previous climate of punitive action has been replaced by a culture of safety and patient care improvement. Administration and staff inquire about what changes are being made to reduce errors. There is a higher percentage of near misses reported compared to actual errors reported, which may confirm this trend toward a culture of safety. It is likely that there are still errors and adverse reactions that occur that are not reported, and the pharmacy and nursing departments continue to work on trying to capture events. Keeping the reporting system in the forefront with staff—by promoting the improvements made and by utilization of the system on a quarterly basis through staff meetings and newsletters—has kept reporting of events and near misses at good levels.

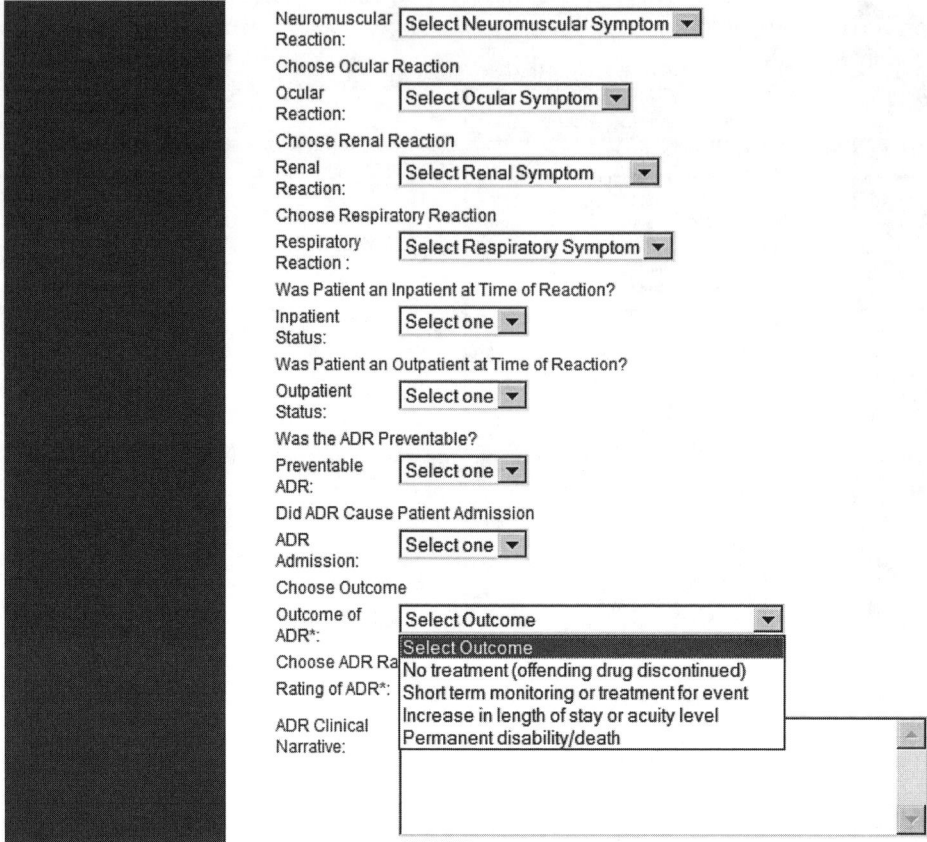

Figure 14.5. Other drop-down boxes include patient admission status, whether the adverse drug reaction was preventable, and whether the reaction caused an admission. Finally, the staff member is asked to choose the outcome of the reaction and rating (mild, moderate, or severe). There is room for a clinical narrative of event as well. By saving the page after entry of all information, the adverse drug reaction is stored in the server database and a notification of the reaction is emailed to the director of pharmacy.

15

Utilizing a Clinical Pharmacist for Refill Triage to Increase Medication Safety in an Internal Medicine Clinic

Ernest J. Dole
Gisela I. Robles
Matthew M. Murawski

Introduction and Rationale for Utilization of Clinical Pharmacist as a Medication Safety Agent

The National Coordinating Council for Medication Error Reporting and Prevention defines a medication error as "any preventable event that may cause or lead to inappropriate medication use or patient harm while the medication is in the control of the healthcare professional, patient, or consumer. Such events may be related to professional practice, healthcare products, procedures, and systems including prescribing; order communication; product labeling, packaging and nomenclature; compounding; dispensing; distribution; administration; education; monitoring; and use."[1]

The 1999 Institute of Medicine (IOM) report, "To Err Is Human: Building a Safer Health System," estimated that 44,000 to 98,000 people die each year from preventable medication errors in U.S. hospitals.[2] Nationwide, the annual cost of drug-related morbidity and mortality in the U.S. is approximately $76 to $136 billion.[3] Therefore, it is reasonable to state that medication errors can cost many lives and a lot of money. How can the addition of a clinical pharmacist to an inpatient clinic setting impact medication safety and decrease medication errors?

The classification of medication errors depends on the severity of the patient outcome (Table 15.1).[4] These categories are No Error (category A); Error and No Harm (categories B through D); Error and Harm (categories E through H), and Error and Death (category I).[4]

Pharmacists are in a unique position to proactively prevent medication errors in categories A and B (near misses), identify potential sources of medication errors in the medication-use process (prescribing, dispensing, and administration of drugs), and can potentially stop medication errors from reaching patients.[5]

Two different hospital studies, conducted by the same primary investigator, were published in *Pharmacotherapy* in 2001 and 2006. Both studies offered evidence supporting the participation of decentralized pharmacy services as impacting the decrease in medication errors. In the first study, Bond and colleagues evaluated factors associated with medication errors and medication errors that affected patient care outcomes in reporting U.S. hospitals (n = 1,116).[6] For all patients admitted yearly to these hospitals, the total medication error rate was 5% with 0.25% of these medication errors having adversely impacted patient outcomes. Factors associated with decreased medication errors included an affiliation with pharmacy teaching programs and decentralized pharmacy services.

Table 15.1. Medication Error Index for Categorizing Errors

Error	Category	Result
No error	A	Circumstances or events that have the capacity to create error
Error, no harm	B	An error occurred but the medication did not reach the patient
	C	An error occurred that reached the patient but did not cause the patient harm
	D	An error occurred that resulted in the need for increased patient monitoring but no patient harm
Error, harm	E	An error occurred that resulted in the need for treatment or intervention and caused temporary patient harm
	F	An error occurred that resulted in initial or prolonged hospitalization and caused temporary patient harm
	G	An error occurred that resulted in permanent patient harm
	H	An error occurred that resulted in a near-death event
Error, death	I	An error occurred that resulted in patient death

Some studies have included adverse drug reactions (ADRs) as medication errors, if the reactions were considered preventable. It is important to mention that some studies use the terms *ADR* and *adverse drug event (ADE)* interchangeably. An ADR is a "response to a drug which is noxious and unintended and which occurs at doses normally used for prophylaxis, diagnosis, or therapy of disease or for the modification of physiologic function while an ADE is an injury resulting from the use of a drug."[7]

In 2006, Bond and Raehl evaluated factors associated with 35,193 ADRs reported in hospitalized Medicare patients at 584 U.S. hospitals. Reductions in ADR rates were significant in hospitals offering pharmacist-provided admission drug histories, drug protocol management, and ADR management. Conversely, for hospitals without pharmacist-provided ADR management, increases in ADR rates, length of stay (14%), death rate (54%), and total Medicare charges (7%) were reported.[8]

To improve medication safety and, more specifically, to optimize noncancer pain medication therapy, a medication safety program utilizing a pharmacist clinician (Ph.C.)* was implemented in an integrated health system in New Mexico. The program goal was to develop policies and procedures, guided by the clinic's collaborative practice agreement for medication safety specific to medications for chronic conditions, including controlled pain medications. Guidelines for medication safety programs are outlined in the "Leading Strategic Planning Effort, Pathways for Medication Safety" document issued by the partnership of the American Hospital Association, Health and Educational Trust and Institute for Safe Medication Practices.[12]

The program specific goals and steps to implementation are outlined below.

---

*In April 1993, the legislature of New Mexico enacted the Pharmacist Prescriptive Authority Act, which granted prescriptive authority to pharmacists designated as Ph.C. In New Mexico a Ph.C. is a registered pharmacist with advanced training in the areas of physical assessment and pharmacotherapy who is eligible for prescriptive authority and enters into a collaborative practice agreement with a supervising physician. The act requires that these clinicians have additional training "at least equivalent to the training of a physician assistant." A Ph.C. with prescriptive authority can prescribe, modify, and monitor drug therapy in accordance with a written protocol registered with the New Mexico Board of Pharmacy.[10,11]

Background and Implementation of the Clinic

The Lovelace Medical Group is a for-profit, integrated health system located in Albuquerque, New Mexico. It includes a health plan (HP), five hospitals, and 14 ambulatory clinics. The Gibson Internal Medicine clinic, part of the Lovelace Medical Group, utilizes one Ph.C., 10 physicians, and one nurse practitioner and serves a patient base of 21,000. Approximately 48% of clinic patients are non-Hispanic white, 48% Hispanic, 2% African-American, and 2% other ethnicities. The average age of patients is 60 years old. The group HP insures 80% of clinic patients.[9] Any provider in the healthcare system may refer patients to the Ph.C. clinic. The clinic was opened in May 2004 and its goals are below:

1. Provide chronic noncancer pain patients with excellent medication therapy management of their condition

2. Decrease liability to clinic providers by centralizing all the controlled substance prescribing

3. Implement a medication safety program utilizing a Ph.C. This program has two components: (1) centralizing all medication refills through the Ph.C. so that irregularities could be quickly spotted and followed up, and (2) centralizing all controlled substance prescribing so patients that could be diverting or using their pain medicines inappropriately can be identified quickly.

4. Provide pharmaceutical care to health-system patients, including patients with stable, chronic diseases who are receiving multiple medications, via collaborative practice agreements with providers in the health system.

5. Improve patient outcomes and decrease adverse effects by controlling polypharmacy (defined as patient concurrently receiving ≥5 medications)

6. Provide a comprehensive patient medication profile and appropriate monitoring parameters

7. Provide the most effective drug regimen possible, in a cost-effective fashion

The Ph.C. sees an average of 18 patients daily, 90% of which are chronic pain patients. The Ph.C. sees patients for 5 hours a day between the hours of 8 a.m. to 11 a.m. and 1 p.m. to 3 p.m. The hours not dedicated to patient care are used for triaging the clinic's refill requests.

A component of the clinic is utilizing the Ph.C. as a medication safety agent. The Ph.C. also triages refills, thus ensuring uniformity of procedures for authorizing refills. Before the implementation of this clinic, there was no standardization of the medication refill process. The medication safety/refill segment of the clinic is now a collaborative practice endeavor between the internal medicine service's medical staff, the Ph.C., and two licensed practical nurses (LPNs). The collaborative practice protocols were developed using National Cholesterol Education Program Adult Treatment Program (NCEP ATP III) guidelines for cholesterol treatment.[13] Veteran Affairs/Department of Defense and the World Health Organization's pain ladder were utilized for development of the chronic pain collaborative practice protocols.[14,15] The New Mexico Board of Pharmacy and the New Mexico Board of Medical Examiners approved the protocols.

The Ph.C., the clinic's nurse clinical coordinator, the supervising physician, and two LPNs developed a pharmacy medication refill protocol. Medication classes and monitoring parameters under the protocol include chronic medications such as thyroid hormone replacement and thyroid stimulating hormone; angiotension converting enzyme inhibitors and blood pressure; serum creatinine and potassium; diabetes mellitus medications and glycosylated hemoglobin; antilipemic agents and NCEP ATP III goals; antihypertensives and JNC VII goals; and central nervous system agents and psychotropic agents filled for 3 months maximum. The protocol also includes medications used in the treatment of chronic nonmalignant pain, such as opioids, muscle relaxants, neuropathic agents, and nonsteroidal anti-inflammatory drugs. A database was developed to track the prescribing of controlled substances. This database included the patient's name, medical record number, referring provider, date of written prescription, name of medication, strength of medication, number of doses, number of days supply, and visual analogue score for pain. (Refill requests for acutely administered medications, such as oral antibiotics, opioid cough syrups, and otic and ophthalmic antibiotics, are referred to the triage nurse for evaluation.)

The LPNs process refill requests by obtaining laboratory values based on medication specific protocols and when the primary provider last saw the patient. The following parameters of this process are tracked: number of refills daily, number of refills per provider/day, number of patients who have not been seen in >1 year, and number of patients with monitoring tests that need to be obtained or rechecked (i.e., "near-miss" events). The success of the medication safety program was measured by the number of "near-miss" medication errors caught. A "near miss" was defined by missed office visits and abnormal laboratory values that were not followed up on in a reasonable time period, such as a patient not being followed up within 6 weeks for an abnormal TSH level, or for a blood pressure not being rechecked 1 month after medication change, or for a patient not being seen in the clinic for greater than 1 year. The clinic also tracked near-miss events that were avoided by Ph.C. triage of medication refills.

Medication Safety/Refill Authorization Results

An average of 150 refill requests/day were processed over the past 3 years. During the same time period, there was an average of 10 patients daily that had not seen their provider in over a year, or who had abnormal laboratory results that were not identified by the patient's primary care provider. The most common abnormal laboratory test needing followup was thyroid-stimulating hormone. Under the collaborative practice protocol utilized in this clinic, the Ph.C. was able to adjust and prescribe medications for chronic nonmalignant pain, order appropriate laboratory tests, and write prescriptions for chronic medications to bridge the patient until the patient was able to see his/her primary care provider. Utilizing a Ph.C. with prescriptive authority to triage and approve medication refill requests has helped streamline the process for patients to obtain medication refills and increase consistency of authorizations

Conclusion

While it is hard to demonstrate the clinical and economic impact of this clinic on medication safety, clinic leadership believes this Gibson clinic medication safety program has increased medication safety among its patient population and resulted in cost savings to health plans. Additionally, as a direct result of the program, a large number of patients were brought back into the clinic for evaluation that would otherwise have been lost to followup.

Over the years medication safety has become a priority in pharmacy practice. It is now recognized that safe medication practices have a direct impact in patient outcomes. Today's pharmacy practitioners proactively seek out and prevent medication errors and ADRs that may arise during the medication-use process. Not only can pharmacists improve the health of patients and protect them from subtherapeutic and/or harmful treatments, but pharmacists can also seek to lower the healthcare costs by avoiding the cost consequences of medication errors and preventable ADRs.

References

1. National Coordinating Council for Medication Error Reporting and Prevention. What is a medication error? Available at: http://www.nccmerp.org/aboutMedErrors.html. Accessed on November 26, 2006.

2. Institute of Medicine of the National Academies. To Err is Human: Building a safer health system. Available at: http://www.iom.edu/CMS/2955.aspx. Accessed November 26, 2006.

3. Johnson JA, Bootman LJ. Drug-related morbidity and mortality: a cost-of-illness model. *Arch Intern Med.* 1995;155:1949-1956.

4. United States Pharmacopeia. National Coordinating Council for Medication Error Reporting and Prevention Index for categorizing medication errors. Available at: http://www.usp.org/patientSafety/medmarx/. Accessed on November 26, 2006.

5. Mangino PD. Role of the pharmacist in reducing medication errors. *J Surg Oncol.* 2004;88:189-194.

6. Bond CA, Raehl CL, Franke T. Medication errors in United States hospitals. *Pharmacotherapy.* 2001;21(9):1023-1036.

7. Nebeker JR, Barach P, Samore MH. Clarifying adverse drug events: A clinician's guide to terminology, documentation, and reporting. *Ann Intern Med.* 2004;140:795-801.

8. Bond CA, Raehl CL. Clinical pharmacy services, pharmacy staffing, and adverse drug reactions in United States hospitals. *Pharmacotherapy.* 2006;26(6):735-747.

9. Parrott T. Opioid analgesics for chronic noncancer pain in primary care. *J Am Board Fam Pract.* 1999;12(4):293-306.

10. Pharmacist scope of practice. American College of Physicians-American Society of Internal Medicine. *Arch Intern Med.* 2002;136:79-85.

11. Dole EJ. Profession of second lieutenants. *Am J Health Syst Pharm.* 2002;59:558-560.

12. Leading a Strategic Planning Effort, Pathways for Medication Safety. A Partnership: American Hospital Association, Health Research and Educational Trust and Institute for Safe Medication Practices. 2002 [cited 2007 Aug 31]. Available from: http://www.medpathways.info.

13. Third report of the national cholesterol education program (NCEP) expert panel on detection, evaluation, and treatment of high blood cholesterol in adults (adult treatment panel III).[monograph on the internet]. Washington: U.S. Department of Health and Human Services; 2002 [cited 2006 Mar 15]. Available from: http://www.nhlbi.nih.gov/guidelines/cholestero/atpsfull.pdf.

14. VHA/DoD clinical practice guidelines for the management of clinically unexplained symptoms: chronic pain and fatigue.{monograph on the internet]. Washington: National Guideline Clearing house; 2001 [cited 2006 Mar 15]. Available from: http://www.guidelines.gov.summary/html.

15. WHO's pain ladder [monograph on the internet]. Geneva, Switzerland: World Health Organization; 2006 (cited 2006 Mar 15). Available from: http://www.who.int/cancer/palliative/painladder/en/.

16

Here Today, Gone Tomorrow! Dealing with Drug Shortages

Agatha L. Nolen

Drug shortages are a fact of life for every hospital, regardless of facility size or patient mix. There are a variety of reasons that drugs shortages occur including raw and bulk material unavailability, manufacturing difficulties, voluntary recalls, manufacturer production decisions, orphan drug products, restricted drug product distribution, industry consolidations, market shifts, unexpected increases in demand, nontraditional distributors, and natural disasters.[1] Some shortages occur with ample notice for action. Other shortages involve drugs with fairly low usage and current stock on hand is adequate until the shortage is resolved. Manufacturers have also increased efforts in recent years to announce when a shortage of drug will occur, and regularly place a limited supply of drug product on an "allocation basis" to qualified customers.

The purpose of this article is to present a case study of a drug shortage in which the drug was one that was critical to patient care, no viable substitute was available, and the drug was placed on an allocation basis directly from the manufacturer.

Background

Centennial Medical Center is a Hospital Corporation of America (HCA) acute-care, 615-bed facility located in Nashville, TN. Principal services include cardiology, oncology, cardiovascular surgery, obstetrics, kidney transplant, and orthopedics. Centennial Medical Center performs over 1,200 cardiac surgery cases per year.*

The therapeutics and infection (T&I) committee is composed of members of the medical staff who meet monthly to review medication use, approve medications for use, and set medication use policy for the hospital. All drug substitutions monographs are prepared by members of the pharmacy staff and approved by the T&I committee. These recommendations are then forwarded to the medical executive committee (MEC) for final approval at their monthly meeting. All medical staff departments are represented on the MEC. Typically these MEC decisions are prepared, reviewed, and approved within a 1-month timeframe, although some decisions are delayed due to a lack of complete information, or agenda items being tabled at one of the MEC meetings due to the length of the agenda. After final approval by the MEC, a communication plan is developed with input from the medical staff, pharmacy, and nursing departments and an implementation date is set. The time from drug substitution monograph preparation and final implementation is typically 6–8 weeks.

---

*The number of cardiac surgery cases was obtained from Centennial Medical Center's departments of Accounting and Coding.

This process is in compliance with the Joint Commission™ standard MM.2.10, "Medications available for dispensing or administration (including stock medications) are selected, listed and procured based on criteria." The elements of performance for MM.2.10 include #7: The hospital has processes to address medication shortages and outages, including the following:

- Communicating with prescribers and staff who participate in the medication management system,
- Developing approved substitution protocols,
- Educating licensed independent practitioners and healthcare staff who participate, in the medication management system about these protocols, and
- Obtaining medications in the event of a disaster."[2]

Because back orders (and consequent shortages) for a particular product are common from Centennial's wholesaler, the pharmacy developed a drug shortage management process for the pharmacy buyer to use on a daily basis. When faced with a back order, the pharmacy buyer follows these steps:

1. Ascertains the current quantity on hand of the back-ordered item to determine if immediate action is required. If an adequate inventory exists until the next routine order, the buyer notes the back order and attempts to place the order for the drug again at the next regularly scheduled order.

2. If an inadequate inventory exists, the buyer reviews alternatives for the same size and strength from a different manufacturer. (The buyer can order the alternative product if the price difference between the normally ordered product and the alternative manufacturer is less than a preset limit.)

3. If the buyer is able to locate the same size and strength from a different manufacturer through the wholesaler, but the cost exceeds the preset spending limit, the buyer obtains purchase authorization from a member of pharmacy management staff.

4. If the buyer is unable to locate the exact size and strength from an alternative manufacturer through the wholesaler, a list of available products of different sizes or strengths is compiled. This list is reviewed by the pharmacy director and clinical coordinator to determine if the substitutions are appropriate for the clinical situations where the product will be used and are not likely to increase the potential for medication errors. If changing the size or strength of a product may cause a medication error, potential ways of mitigating the risk (e.g., repackaging of the product, removing from floor stock, issuing the drug on a per patient basis only) are evaluated. Often, nursing administration and physicians who routinely use the drug are consulted for this evaluation prior to the purchase.

5. Other local institutions are then consulted to determine if the shortage is isolated to one wholesaler or manufacturer. Often, other facilities who utilize different purchasing entities can loan a small amount of product until the shortage has abated through normal channels. Centennial does not use 3rd-party resellers and only purchases products through its traditional wholesalers.

6. If no product is available in any size or strength that is equivalent, a review of all uses of the product in short supply is conducted by the clinical pharmacy staff. Each clinician reviews

the product's indications and usage and recommends an appropriate alternative. The clinician works directly with the buyer to determine if alternatives are available and in adequate supply.

7. After all reviews are conducted, they are presented to the pharmacy management team for input. After recommendations are finalized, they are presented at the next T&I committee and MEC for approval and implementation.

This is Centennial's typical process when dealing with a drug shortage. What happens when a drug shortage occurs on too short notice to utilize the normal committee structure for decision-making? What happens when the drug in short supply can not be substituted with another product and is used in a prominent product line of the hospital?

The following case study illustrates what happens when a critical drug shortage is not handled appropriately at the outset.

Case Study

Tuesday, 1300:

The Centennial pharmacy buyer notifies the director of pharmacy and the clinical coordinator that all strengths of protamine are unavailable from the wholesaler. The pharmacy director knows that protamine is used in cardiac surgery cases and that the facility does approximately 1,200 cases per year.* The pharmacy buyer is directed to execute the drug shortage management plan.

Tuesday, 1400:

The pharmacy director receives a call from the cardiology pharmacist who has just heard that the pharmacy is unable to obtain protamine. The pharmacy director indicates that the pharmacy is working on the shortage and will notify him when a plan has been developed.

Tuesday, 1500:

The cardiology pharmacist contacts the pharmacy director with information that he has shared the "potential" protamine shortage with the chief of the Department of Cardiac Surgery.

Tuesday, 1530:

The pharmacy director retrieves voicemail from the assistant administrator for cardiac product line. The administrator has just received a personal visit from the chief of cardiac surgery demanding to know if all cardiac surgery cases for the following day should be cancelled due to protamine unavailability.

Tuesday, 1540:

The pharmacy director contacts the assistant administrator and the chief of cardiac surgery and tells them that Centennial still has protamine available and that no cardiac surgery cases should be cancelled for the next day. In addition, the pharmacy director indicates he will have a complete report for them by 0900 the next morning with an update on the protamine shortage.

---

*The number of cardiac surgery cases was obtained from Centennial Medical Center's departments of Accounting and Coding.

Tuesday, 1545:

The pharmacy director assembles the pharmacy buyer, clinical coordinator, pharmacy technician supervisor, and cardiology pharmacist in the office. Everyone is instructed that there are to be no more communications to anyone in the hospital on the protamine shortage until further notice. Assignments are made as follows with directions to bring all the requested information to a 0700 meeting the next morning:

Pharmacy Buyer

"Find out how much protamine we have on hand. Count everything and don't forget that we have satellite pharmacies, outpatient areas, drugs trays/carts/kits, disaster drugs, drugs pulled with short (but not expired) dating…even look under your desk!"

"Call the protamine manufacturer directly to confirm the shortage. Find out the exact status of the shortage and when drug will be available. If an allocation program exists, be prepared to tell us what the rules for allocation are.

Also tell us if there are any local facilities that can loan us product until we can obtain more."

Clinical Coordinator/Cardiology Pharmacist

"Find out where we're using protamine. Is protamine being used for any indications where we can substitute another drug? Is there a way to modify the surgical procedures to use less drug? What is the timeframe for the next T&I meeting?"

Pharmacy Technician Supervisor

"Run reports from unit-based cabinets to see how much protamine we have on hand, and what the usage is."

Wednesday, 0700:

Everyone is assembled in the conference room for the management meeting.

- **Where is the drug?** The pharmacy buyer and technician supervisor report first. There is protamine in the main pharmacy, OR pharmacy, open heart carts in main surgery, and tackle boxes in day surgery and women's surgery. Based on current usage Centennial has approximately a 2-week supply of the drug.

- **When do we get more?** The buyer reports that all local facilities are reporting a similar shortage and no one can loan Centennial product. The buyer also reports that based on a direct call to the manufacturer, the product will be in short supply for an unknown duration and the manufacturer has established an allocation procedure. The manufacturer stated that the allocation process for protamine is that each wholesaler account is permitted to order five vials of protamine per week. The pharmacy director asks, "Did I understand correctly? Is the allocation based 'per' wholesaler account?" The answer is, "Yes, it is five vials per wholesaler account."

- **How can Centennial maximize its allocation without stockpiling drugs?** Based on the allocation schema as developed by the manufacturer, Centennial was able to calculate out its patient needs for cardiac surgery cases and continue to supply the needed drug without interruption and without delays or cancellations of cardiac surgery cases. In response to the shortage, Centennial used two previously established dietary and materials management wholesaler accounts in addition to its primary drug wholesaler account, all at the same delivery address but with different delivery locations. A quick phone call to the wholesaler confirmed that there were no restrictions on the number of accounts, and that protamine could be ordered through all three accounts resulting in 15 vials of protamine per week.

However, based on the number of cardiac surgery cases typically performed each week, Centennial still needed more protamine. A call to two sister hospitals in Nashville confirmed that although these facilities did not perform cardiac surgery cases, they were eligible to order protamine from the same wholesaler. These two hospitals began ordering their weekly allocation of protamine and immediately sent it to Centennial Medical Center upon arrival each Monday.

- ***Next question: How to communicate the plan?*** The management team devised a communication scheme, which was comprehensive because of the concern that cardiac surgery cases would need to be cancelled or a serious patient event could occur if the pharmacy ran out of protamine. In order to allay any fears, a comprehensive count was made of all protamine vials on hand and the estimated "days supply" calculated based on the average number of cardiac surgery cases performed each week. This grid included the current day's date, number of protamine vials on hand, and estimated day's supply, and it was updated every morning after arrival of the morning wholesaler order. This grid was posted in the main pharmacy, the OR satellite pharmacy, and the main scheduling board in the main OR. The pharmacy buyer was responsible for updating the information and confirming supplies on hand.

Wednesday, 0900:

The director of pharmacy meets with the assistant administrator, chairman of the T&I committee, and the chief of cardiac surgery. He describes the pharmacy's plan to address the protamine shortage as follows: "Gentlemen, I have good news for you. Based on a closer review, we have adequate protamine to continue to perform cardiac surgery cases at our current volumes. To assure you and your colleagues that this is the case, we will daily post our inventory levels and estimated day's supply at the scheduling board in the main OR and OR pharmacy so that everyone is aware of the current situation. If at any time, you have any further questions, do not hesitate to contact me directly by pager. We will also be sending out a communication to all nursing staff and members of the medical staff as well as posting a notification in the doctors' dining room explaining the nationwide shortage, what we have done to remedy it for our patients, and our ongoing communication plan."

Discussion

Typically, in a shortage situation wholesaler-based drug allocation procedures have certain rules that qualify facilities to participate. Common allocation protocols include reviews of historical purchases, allocations per patient type, and per facility based on physical address.

Centennial felt justified in requesting its two sister facilities to order protamine even though those facilities did not have cardiac surgery programs because Centennial had a legitimate patient need for the protamine and was not stockpiling the allocations. Close tracking of protamine inventory and usage allowed Centennial to cancel orders at its sister facilities during weeks with a lower number of cardiac surgery cases.

In managing drug shortages it is important to obtain accurate information about both the details of the shortage, as well as current and projected usage.

Accurate information on the shortage begins the process. Typically, Centennial contacts the manufacturer directly to determine when the end of the shortage is predicted, the rules of any allocation programs, and if direct ordering is possible.

Accurate information on current usage is also critical. Clinicians should immediately review all current, in-house usage of a product in short supply to determine if any substitutions are acceptable alternatives. Any alternatives that are considered must be evaluated for potential patient safety risks when changing a manufacturer, active ingredient, strength, or dosage form. Once a plan to address the shortage is developed, having preplanned decision-makers identified is also essential. When critical drug shortages occur on short notice, it may be impossible to wait for the next round of formal, medical staff committee meetings to occur. It is important to identify who in your medical staff or administration can authorize an emergency substitution without full committee approval.

Once a plan is developed, organized and calm communication is important to a smooth execution. It is often necessary to use multiple modalities when communicating a critical drug shortage to the pharmacy, nursing, and medical staffs. Centennial uses combinations of the following approaches in getting information to medical staffs:

- Phone calls to physicians with patients affected by the shortage
- Phone calls to department chairs when the drug is primarily used by one group of physicians (e.g., Protonix shortage—GI subcommittee)
- Clinical pharmacy staff contact of 10 key physicians on their services
- "Special Communications" bulletin posted in main pharmacy and other appropriate locations such as the main OR scheduling board and OR satellite pharmacies
- E-mail to physicians' distribution lists
- Formularies on personal digital assistants (PDAs)
- Flyers in the doctors' dining room
- Formulary comments in the computerized provider order entry (CPOE) system

Centennial often utilizes similar modalities, such as e-mail and "Special Communications," to provide information to its pharmacists. In addition "walking in-services" are used for pharmacy and nursing staff members who are unable to assemble in a central location for information sharing. Centennial also attaches formulary comments or blocks order entry in the pharmacy computer system when drugs are in short supply or unavailable. These steps are particularly important for remote order-entry sites where it is not a simple matter of "checking the shelf" for inventory availability when order entry is being done miles from the patient's location.

For nurses, comments are included in our electronic medication administration (eMAR) record so substitution information or patient restrictions are available each time nurses administer the drug or receive an order.

Another important, but often overlooked, communication tool is to post information about the shortage at the main inventory storage site of the product itself. This step is especially important for the main storage location, which is where the staff is most likely to go when receiving a phone call from another facility to "borrow" a drug. The main inventory should clearly be marked with the "rules" to loan the drug out: who can it be loaned to, how is it returned, and any special authorizations (e.g., the pharmacy director). In some cases, special patient criteria are developed through the T&I committee to ensure appropriate use. These criteria should be posted as well and may be utilized to determine when a facility in critical need may borrow a drug. Ensuring that the patient of the borrowing facility meets your internal criteria will maximize a limited supply for everyone. One of the worst situations is to have a drug in short supply and check the shelf in the morning only to find out that the night pharmacist didn't have time to read his e-mail and loaned the entire stock of the drug to another hospital in the middle of the night!

Also, don't forget to communicate after the crisis is over. In fact, routine communications are more effective. At Centennial, the T&I committee and MEC receive a monthly status report of all current drug shortages and remedies. This strategy ensures committee members have accurate information when asked about drug shortage rumors from other members of the medical staff. Ideally, a quarterly report, or at a minimum an annual report, should be presented to the hospital board of directors. The board of directors should understand the safety issues that surround drug shortages and be aware of actions taken by the pharmacy department in conjunction with the medical staff committees to protect the safety of their patients when drug shortages occur.

When faced with critical drug shortages, four elements are crucial: 1) a uniform process that is established well in advance; 2) authority for all steps in the process is outlined in hospital policies and procedures and medical staff bylaws; 3) everyone knows their role; and 4) everyone with a "need to know," knows!

References

1. American Society of Health-System Pharmacists. ASHP guidelines on managing drug product shortages. *Am J Health Syst Pharm*. 2001;58:1445-1450.
2. *Comprehensive Accreditation Manual for Hospitals: The Official Handbook (CAMH)*. Oak Brook Terrace, IL: Joint Commission on Accreditation of Healthcare Organizations; 2006.

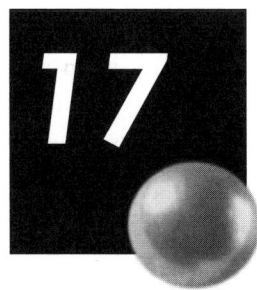

Latex Isn't a Drug—
Why Should I Care?

Connie Larson

Acknowledgments: The author recognizes the contributions of Peggy Bickham, Pharm.D., and the latex allergy task force at the University of Illinois Medical Center at Chicago.

Institution Background

The University of Illinois Medical Center located in Chicago, Illinois, is a 464-bed, tertiary care, academic medical center providing medical and surgical services. The organization's safety structure includes the following committees: pharmacy and therapeutics (P&T), safety, and the medication system review committee (MSRC). MSRC is a subcommittee of P&T and has regular reporting responsibilities to both the P&T and safety committees. The medication safety officer, a role filled by a pharmacist, is the chair of MSRC. The medication safety officer sets the agenda for MSRC meetings and coordinates committee activities. MSRC is charged with ensuring the safety of the medication-use system within the University of Illinois Medical Center. MSRC regularly reviews identified internal safety concerns and outside resources (e.g., *ISMP Medication Safety Alert!*) to proactively address potential problems.

MSRC received a concern from a pharmacist noting problems in identifying patients with latex allergies at the medical center. The pharmacist's prior experience at another hospital involved a patient death related to latex allergy at the medical center. Although patient allergies were documented in the medical record, the pharmacy did not consistently acknowledge latex allergies. As a result, pharmacy personnel did not always use the proper procedures to prepare medications for patients with latex allergies.

Prior to 2006, the practice at the medical center was to question patients about allergies or sensitivities in general. Allergies, including latex allergy or sensitivity, were then recorded by entering the appropriate data into the allergy section of the patient's electronic medical record (EMR). The EMR has a computerized prescriber order entry (CPOE) system that interfaces with the pharmacy computer system and both systems have drug-allergy interaction checking capability. However, given that latex is not a drug, the system does not provide a drug-allergy alert. The result was that even though patients coming into the facility had a properly documented latex allergy, it was often overlooked by the prescriber and the pharmacy. MSRC decided to assemble a group to review this issue in more depth. A latex allergy task force was formed and charged by the MSRC to review the identified problem and develop practical solutions to bring back for committee approval.

Task Force Development

The interdisciplinary latex allergy task force formed included representatives from the materials management, food service, and housekeeping departments, and a variety of inpatient clinical areas representing nursing units and procedural areas (e.g., radiology and surgical services). The chairperson for the committee was the pharmacy operations manager. The pharmacy medication safety technician assisted the group by arranging meetings, taking minutes, distributing handouts, and participating in meeting discussions. The first step for the task force was to educate its members on the scope of the problem and reinforce the importance of the initiative before attempting any process review.

Problem Review and Group Preparation

Latex allergy is an IgE-mediated reaction to natural latex rubber, found in many products and medical supplies. Latex allergies can have a significant negative impact on an individual. The incidence of latex allergy in the general population has been estimated at 1% to 6%.[1-3] Healthcare workers have been identified by the Occupational Safety and Health Administration (OSHA), Centers for Disease Control and Prevention (CDC), and professional associations as being at increased risk (8% to 17%) of developing a sensitivity or allergy to natural latex.[4,5] Another at risk group is latex industry workers. Latex sensitization or allergy in latex industry and healthcare workers has resulted in chronic illness, disability, career loss, hardship, and death. Development of latex sensitivity or allergy of any severity level can occur without warning after many years of uneventful exposure.

The allergic reaction an individual may experience may be an allergic contact dermatitis or an immediate hypersensitivity reaction, ranging in severity from contact urticaria to rapidly progressing systemic anaphylaxis and death. Once sensitized, there is no treatment except for complete avoidance of latex.

Development of Project Goals

To improve patient and employee safety, it is necessary to minimize the risk of exposure, sensitization, and allergic reaction to latex-containing products. Identification of individuals and groups (Table 17.1) with "at risk" characteristics is helpful so these individuals can be specifically questioned to determine sensitization status.

It is important in the healthcare environment to follow the guidelines below in order to minimize patient and employee contact with and exposure to natural latex rubber:

- Implement safe procedures for the care of patients with a known allergy to latex.
- Use only latex-free gloves and supplies when caring for latex-allergic patients.

Table 17.1. Latex Allergy and Sensitivity Risk Factors

At-Risk Individual Characteristics	At-Risk Groups
Past reactions to latex	Healthcare workers
Spina bifida	Latex industry workers
Genitourinary anomalies	
Neurological impairments	
Multiple surgeries	
Repeated or chronic intravenous and urinary catheterizations	
Cross-reactive food allergies	
Bananas, avocado, celery, fig, chestnut, papaya, kiwi, passion fruit	

- Minimize latex allergen environmental contamination by purchasing latex-free products whenever such products are available and suitable for intended use.

- Ensure that employees with potential latex sensitivity or allergy are referred to the facilities' employee access health services for evaluation and recommendations.

- Provide reasonable accommodations for employees with latex sensitivity or allergy.

- Allow only mylar balloons in the care environments.

Internal Assessment—Review of Current Systems

The group decided that the biggest problem at The University of Illinois Medical Center was that products, including medical supplies (e.g., gloves, syringes, catheters) and medications, were purchased with no thought as to their latex content. The group reviewed all purchased medical supplies to determine the products that contained latex and investigated suitable nonlatex alternatives to eliminate latex products from the workplace as much as possible. Once implemented, this step made direct caregivers' jobs much easier, since they weren't constantly trying to find appropriate (latex-free) products for latex-allergic patients. It also minimized caregiver exposure to latex, thus decreasing their risk of developing latex allergy.

For the pharmacy, the task force found that ensuring proper medication preparation for patients with latex allergies was "hit or miss," since the latex allergy could easily be overlooked. At the time of this review, when latex-allergic patients were identified it was common practice for pharmacy personnel to remove the rubber stoppers from vials containing medication for injection, thus eliminating the potential for a needle to introduce latex into the medication vial during the preparation of a patient's IV medication. Review of the literature found two key articles[6,7] that questioned the value of removing the medication vial stopper in latex-allergic patients. The necessity of removing the stopper was discussed with the pharmacy management group, and following a survey of practice at other medical centers, the pharmacy decided to eliminate this step.

Action Plan

The task force, focusing on the problem from a patient safety perspective, looked at all avenues to alert the front-line caregivers to be constantly vigilant while taking care of patients with latex allergies. In particular, nurses, as the most direct caregivers, need as many reminders as possible since they predominantly select medical supplies to be used in the care of the patient. From a pharmacy perspective, one could question why pharmacy personnel need to know or care if identification of patients with latex allergies doesn't trigger any special medication preparation procedures. The task force discovered that one way the pharmacy could assist is by providing an alert about patients' latex allergies via the medication label since most patients have medication or IV orders. However, because pharmacy awareness of latex allergies was minimal at best, it would be difficult for the staff to consistently input this information manually into the pharmacy computer system to print on the labels. The task force considered how best to let the system notify caregivers outside of the usual allergy alert mechanism, that was found to be inadequate for nondrug allergies.

Now, as a result of the task force's efforts, all documented latex allergies trigger an automatic header to all medication and large volume intravenous product labels. The label information notes, "LATEX ALLERGY PRECAUTIONS" (Figures 17.1 and 17.2). This action serves to widely distribute this critical information and alleviates the need for a pharmacist to remember to input the information into each medication order.

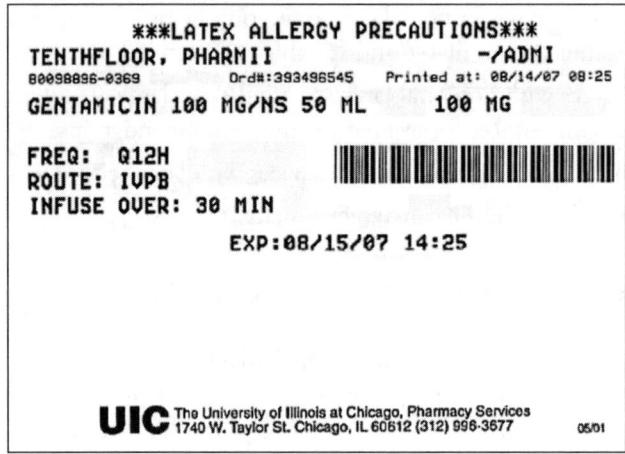

Figure 17.1. Pharmacy Infusion Label Noting Latex Allergy Precautions.

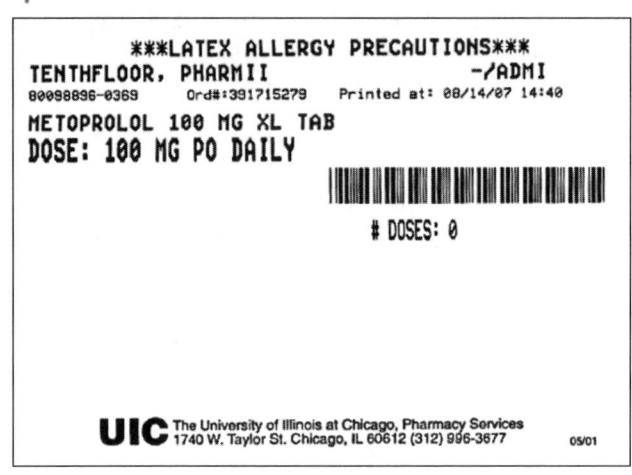

Figure 17.2. Pharmacy Medication Label Noting Latex Allergy Precautions.

Several other strategies were implemented by the task force. Pharmacy and materials management reviewed crash-cart contents and replaced all latex-containing products with latex-free products. The pharmacy is responsible for stocking a latex allergy emergency kit in the automated medication cabinet (AMC) and emergency drug boxes located in the patient care areas. The kit consists of injectable epinephrine 1 mg/mL, 1-mL ampule, diphenhydramine 50 mg/mL, 1-mL vial, and methylprednisolone 62.5 mg/mL, 2-mL vial. The documentation of the latex allergy in the EMR triggers two nursing orders on the patient care plan. Both orders are placed utilizing the medical center's chief medical officer as the prescriber. The first is a nursing order for the latex allergy emergency kit to be "on call PRN" (Figure 17.3). The second nursing order that was implemented directs the nurse to perform key elements* (*see below) of the nursing requirements detailed in the comprehensive policy. Nursing responsibilities start at the admission process and are critical since the documentation of the allergy triggers many of the safety strategies. The specific requirements include the following:

- Inquire if the patient has a latex allergy or sensitivity. (Documentation forms were updated to specifically ask for the information.)

| ☎ | Latex Allergy Emergency Kit | Ordered | 1 EA, KIT, MISC, ON CALL PRN, For Latex Allergic Reaction, Routine, First Dose 03/08/06 15:09:00 |
| ☑ | | | See kit for dosing and administration guidelines; kits are located in the automated medication cabinet and the drug box. Each kit contains 1 vial each of epinephrine, diphenhydramine, and methylprednisolone. Standing order approved by Chief Medical Officer |

Figure 17.3. Medication Order Generated Automatically when Latex Allergy Detected.

- *If so, apply the yellow *latex sensitive* bracelet.
- Document a codified latex allergy that allows the allergy to be recognized (and triggers pharmacy medication label note and nursing orders) on the allergy screen in the EMR, and *place a yellow *latex allergy* sticker on the front of the chart.
- *Post the *latex allergy* sign on the patient's door and above the bed.
- Use only latex-free products (refer to product package labeling). If a latex-free product is not available, provide a barrier between the patient and the item.
- Follow all latex sensitive precautions:
  - ◆ Wash hands prior to entering the patient's room.
  - ◆ Monitor the patient for signs of an allergic reaction.
  - ◆ If necessary, access the latex allergy emergency kit (containing epinephrine, diphenhydramine, and methylprednisolone) kept in the automated medication cabinet and the emergency drug box.
  - ◆ Place latex-allergic patients in rooms away from the supply area.

- If the latex-allergic patient must leave the area for a test or is being transferred, the nurse must perform the following:
  - ◆ Notify the receiving department of the patient's latex allergy.
  - ◆ Ensure the yellow *latex allergy* bracelet is in place.
  - ◆ Ensure that the yellow *latex allergy* sticker is on the front of the patient's chart prior to the patient leaving the unit.
  - ◆ Provide the patient/family with information regarding latex sensitivity/allergy prior to the patient's discharge.
  - ◆ Document that latex allergy precautions were followed during patient care and specify the nonlatex-containing products provided.

Other department initiatives included the dietary department using only latex-free gloves and utensils for food preparation and handling. Also, the housekeeping department agreed to avoid the use of latex-containing gloves and cleaning products. It is easy to enforce these initiatives if latex-containing products, particularly latex gloves, are not purchased at all.

The surgical and procedural areas (e.g., radiology) reviewed their processes to address accommodating patients with latex allergies. Improvements initiated for these areas are below:

- Establishing a system of advance notification of latex-allergic patient for surgical and procedural areas
- Making reasonable attempt to schedule these patients as the first case of the day
- For certain items, the most suitable product for general use is a latex-containing product; for

these items, maintain a supply of latex-free products to be used in the care of latex-allergic patients

Staff Education

A medical center policy was developed, reviewed, and approved by MSRC, P&T, and safety committees. The medical staff executive committee also reviewed and approved the policy. The policy highlights were distributed via email to the medical center staff. Additional education took place at pharmacy and nursing meetings to focus on new processes that impacted their work.

Monitoring

Monitoring the program is facilitated by system reports that are generated by pharmacy personnel from the EMR. Patients that are currently admitted to the hospital are listed along with their documented latex allergies. The medication safety officer monitors the reports and double-checks that the system automated nursing orders and medication label notes are generated appropriately. Compliance has been consistently 100% with no system problems since implementation. Compliance for the intervention steps, placement of the allergy sticker, and placement of the yellow latex allergy bracelet are routinely 100% as collected on a monthly basis, although latex-allergic patients are in-house relatively infrequently (i.e., 1–2 per month).

Summary

The group as a whole thought the project and ultimate policy development was a worthwhile endeavor since the members were not only improving patient care, but also creating a safer environment for the staff. The most effective improvement by far was removing latex-containing products in the workplace where a suitable latex-free option was available. This action made it easier to care for these patients, eliminating the need to request special products from materials management and lessened latex exposure to the staff. The intervention steps that were implemented are effective because the nurse's computer-generated patient task list contains the latex allergy intervention orders as orders to be carried out; nurses do not have to remember steps detailed in a policy. Implementing system improvements based on automation instead of relying on staff to remember policy requirements is a reliable method to enable staff to care for latex-allergic patients.

References

1. Turjanmaa K, Makinen-Kilijunen S, Reunala T, et al. Natural rubber latex allergy: the European experience. *Immunol Allergy Clin North Am.* 1995;15:71-78.
2. Liss GM, Sussman GL. Latex sensitization: occupation versus general population prevalence rates. *Am J Ind Med.* 1999;35:196-200.
3. Bernardini R, Novembre E, Ingargiola A, et al. Prevalence and risk factors of latex sensitization in an unselected pediatric population. *J Allergy Clin Immunol.* 1998;101:621-625.
4. Kaczmarek R, Hamilton RG, Gross TP, et al. Prevalence of latex-specific IgE antibodies in hospital personnel. *Ann Allergy Asthma Immunol.* 1996;76:51-56.
5. Lagier F, Vervloet D, Lhermet I, et al. Prevalence of latex allergy in operating room nurses. *J Allergy Clin Immunol.* 1992;90:319-322.

6. Thomsen DJ, Burke TG. Lack of latex contamination of solutions withdrawn from vials with natural rubber stoppers. *Am J Health Syst Pharm.* 2000;57:44-47.

7. Hamilton RG, Brown RH, Veltri MA, et al. Administering pharmaceuticals to latex-allergic patients from vials containing natural rubber latex closures. *Am J Health Syst Pharm.* 2005;62:1822-1827.

Other Resources

American Latex Allergy Association: http://www.latexallergyresources.org

American Nurses Association: Position Statement, Latex Allergy. http://nursingworld.org/MainMenuCategories/HealthcareandPolicyIssues/ANAPositionStatements/workplac/wklatex14544.aspx. September 15, 1997.

Don't Let Your Patients Fall by the Wayside!

Meghan F. Wilkosz

Acknowledgments: The author recognizes the contributions of Lydia Borysiuk, Robin Harding, Amy Huie-Li, Brian Kotansky, Annette Lipinski, Jennifer McDonald, Bogdan Musial, Kathleen O'Neil, Sadiann Ozment, Mindy Sonet, and Charlie Waters. Each person is affiliated with the VA Connecticut Healthcare System, with the exception of Brian Kotansky, who is affiliated with Z-Consulting, LLC, Meriden, Connecticut.

Introduction to VA Connecticut

The safety Pearl presented in this chapter was created by members of the pharmacy staff at the VA Connecticut Healthcare System (VA CT), West Haven campus, in conjunction with staff from nursing, medical, and physical/occupational therapy as an interdisciplinary team. VA CT West Haven is a government hospital with 211 inpatient beds for patients on general medicine, surgery, geriatrics, psychiatry, and blind rehabilitation services. As one might suspect within a veterans hospital, the patient population consists predominantly of elderly male patients. Hospital staff cares for 50,000 eligible veterans in Connecticut and surrounding areas. The facility also offers numerous specialty services, further expanding the patient population.

Goal of Safety Pearl

The goal of this Pearl is to evaluate a pharmacy medication-review consult service as part of a fall-risk reduction program in an acute care setting in an effort to improve safety in the veteran population. This Pearl describes an interdisciplinary, fall-risk reduction program, including its implementation and evaluation in an effort to address Joint Commission™ patient safety goals.

Definition of Falls and Near Falls

For the purpose of this investigation, a *fall* was defined as a sudden, unintentional change in position causing an individual to land at a lower level, on an object, the floor, or the ground. A *near fall* was defined as a sudden loss of balance not causing a fall or other injury.[1]

Risks and Consequences of Falls

Unfortunately, falls are the leading accidental cause of death due to for older patients ≥65 years of age.[2] Over three-quarters of nursing home residents are expected to fall each year.[2] One of the most devastating consequences of a fall is hip fractures.[3] Once a patient does experience a hip fracture, the mortality rate is approximately 20% within the first 12 months.[4] Patients that fall once have a 50% risk of falling again within the next 12 months.[5]

Numerous factors have been associated with falls. Predisposing risk factors for falls are those that are inherent to the patient's health status. These items are unable to be changed. On the other hand, precipitating risk factors are generally considered environmental in nature and are amenable for intervention. In some cases, medications are a predisposing factor, as some medications are absolutely necessary for appropriate therapy. On the other hand, some medications are a precipitating factor, and changes to the medication regimen can be made in an effort to reduce risk of falling. A table including predisposing and precipitating risk factors is contained in Table 18.1.[6]

In addition to the numerous factors that can cause falls, there are also many consequences related to falls. The consequences of falls, especially in the elderly, are well known and include increased morbidity and mortality, decreased functional status, loss of independence, decreased quality of life, and increased healthcare costs.[5]

Joint Commission Patient Safety Goals and VA National Center for Patient Safety

The Joint Commission has identified patient safety goals for 2006 and 2007 aimed at reducing the risk of harm resulting from patient falls. Goal 9 asks that healthcare systems implement a fall reduction program and evaluate the effectiveness of the program.[7]

In addition to Joint Commission guidance, the VA National Center for Patient Safety (VA NCPS) produced a Falls Toolkit in 2004. The toolkit provides information on designing a falls prevention and management program; implementing effective interventions for high-risk fall patients; using hip protectors for high-risk fall patients; and educating patients, families, and staff on falls and fall injury prevention. The VA NCPS identified falls as an area of intervention because in 2003, falls represented nearly 47% of all safety reports within the VA NCPS database, and falls were involved in 11% of all root cause analyses.[8]

VA Connecticut Falls Policy

In the summer of 2005, an interdisciplinary, falls-risk reduction team was created to develop a hospital policy at VA CT to address the Joint Commission's goal of reducing patient harm resulting from falls. The group decided that the fall prevention program would have two goals: (1) ensuring

Table 18.1. Patient Risk Factors Associated with Falls

Predisposing Risk Factors	Precipitating Risk Factors
Orthostasis	Room obstacles
Arthritis	Furniture
Acute illness	IV poles
Cognitive impairment	Electrical cords
Vision impairment	Loose carpet
Altered gait	
Bowel/bladder urgency	
Loss of muscle strength	

MEDICATIONS

that patients in all care settings are assessed for fall risk, and (2) providing appropriate, preventive environmental and procedural interventions to avoid falls and prevent injuries. Communication among caregivers about the management of patients to prevent falls or the recurrence of falls is an essential component of the program. Any inpatient assessed by the admitting nurse as being at high risk for a fall is identified with a green wrist bracelet, and orange stickers graphically representing fall risk are placed outside the patient's door. The bracelet and sticker communicate the patient's fall risk to staff who can then help the patient by taking the necessary fall precautions.[9]

This policy created an interdisciplinary team to help address the growing issue of falls. Each specialist on the team fills an important role in reducing falls. Physicians serve to evaluate medical history for increased fall risk and implement interventions recommended by other team members. Nurses ensure compliance with fall prevention interventions, while physical therapists evaluate patients for gait, balance, range of motion, and muscle strength via an electronic consult request. Finally, pharmacists are responsible for reviewing medication regimens, per consultation request, and notifying providers about perceived potential negative effects of medications or drug interactions on a patient's fall risk.

In addition to identifying the key players as necessary members of the interdisciplinary team to reduce fall risk, VA CT identified several specific steps that can reduce fall risk, including communication of fall risk and necessary interventions among caregivers; communication of fall risk to patient; evaluation of the physical environment and the patient's ability to ambulate; an assessment of the current safety measures in place; and an evaluation of medical history and medication regimen.

At hospital admission and transfer, the nurse completes a note in a given patient's electronic medical record, including evaluation of the patient's risk for falling. In addition, any time a fall or near fall occurs, a similar post-fall progress note is completed by the nurse caring for the patient. Both the initial and post-fall notes include the patient's baseline functional status, physical status, pain assessment, and, finally, fall risk. Based on this evaluation of the patient's status, the nurse is responsible for ordering consults and implementing interventions appropriate for each patient.

Morse Fall Scale

One essential component of the nurse's note is the Morse Fall Scale (MFS). The MFS is used widely in acute care settings, both in hospital and long-term care facilities. The MFS requires a systematic, reliable assessment of a patient's fall risk factors upon admission, fall, change in health status, or transfer to a new care setting. Components taken into consideration with the MFS are history of falls, secondary diagnosis associated with falls, use of ambulatory aids, IV or heparin locks, gait/transferring status, and mental status. The MFS is included in Table 18.2.[10]

Each individual component of the MFS is given a point score, and all the values are added together to give a final score. The significance of the MFS scores is summarized in Table 18.3.[7] The patient's cumulative MFS score determines the type of fall interventions that are instituted for a given patient.

Medication Use and Falls

An essential component of risk for falls that is not included in the MFS is medication use. Pharmacists recognize that elders are at increased risk of adverse drug events, including falls. For this reason, the original pharmacy fall-risk policy developed at VA CT required that pharmacy consults be requested if patients were on certain classes of medications, as well as documentation of certain symptoms that could be associated with falls. The medication classes considered at VA CT to increase

Table 18.2. Morse Fall Scale (MFS)

Risk Factor	Scale	Score
History of falls	Yes	25
	No	0
Secondary diagnosis	Yes	15
	No	0
Ambulatory aids used	Furniture	30
	Crutches/cane/walker	15
	None/bed rest/wheelchair/nurse	0
IV/heparin lock	Yes	20
	No	0
Gait/transferring	Impaired	20
	Weak	10
	Normal/bed rest/immobile	0
Mental status	Forgets limitations	15
	Oriented to own ability	0

Sum total of the items above =

Table 18.3. Risk Stratification of Morse Fall Scale

Risk Level	MFS Score	Action
No risk	0–24	None
Low risk	25–50	Standard fall prevention interventions
High risk	≥51	High fall prevention interventions

patients' fall risk are presented in Table 18.4. These medications were chosen based on numerous literature references.[11-14]

Symptoms Associated with Falls

In addition to recognizing that certain medications put patients at risk for falling, the multidisciplinary team identified symptoms that are also commonly associated with falls (Table 18.5).

As mentioned previously, nurses are responsible for entering a note evaluating each patient's status when he is admitted, transferred, or has a fall/near fall. This nursing note (called the *intake/reassessment note*) also includes an evaluation of the patient's fall risk, as measured by the MFS. Additionally, nurses are asked to make appropriate interventions based on the patient's fall risk, including consulting physical therapy, implementing environmental fall precautions, and finally, ordering a pharmacy fall-risk consult. The environmental fall precautions that nurses are responsible for implementing and documenting are included in Figure 18.1.

Table 18.4. Medications Commonly Associated with Falls

Cardiac medications
Antihypertensives
Diuretics
Antipsychotics
Hypnotics
Sedating antidepressants
Anticholinergics
Anxiolytics
NSAIDs
Narcotic analgesics
Anticonvulsants
Oral hypoglycemics
Insulin

Table 18.5. Symptoms Commonly Associated with Falls

Dizziness
Orthostatic hypotension
Rigidity
Altered gait
Altered balance
Bowel urgency
Bladder urgency
Change in mentation
Drowsiness

Pharmacist Intervention

In the original fall-risk reduction policy, the clinical pharmacist review of a patient's medication regimen was initiated via a consult request entered by a nurse, based on a patient's predicted risk of falling as evidenced by medication regimen and presenting symptoms. In addition to making general recommendations based on medication classes, clinical pharmacists also made patient-specific recommendations.

In many cases, recommendations were as simple as recommending medication hold parameters if blood pressure, heart rate, or blood sugar were low in patients on antihypertensives, cardiac medications, hypoglycemics, or insulin, respectively. Often, pharmacists recommended decreasing doses or discontinuing medications associated with falls. For example, patients on terazosin for benign prostatic hypertrophy could be changed to tamsulosin, which as a α_{1a}- selective alpha blocker, is less likely to cause hypotension and subsequent falls. Similarly, patients with renal insufficiency and pain could be changed from morphine to a hepatically metabolized drug like oxycodone. Morphine can accumulate in renal insufficiency and cause excessive sedative effects, which could also lead to falls.

Pharmacists also evaluated medications that could cause serious complications if patients administered these medications were to fall, such as aspirin, warfarin, or clopidogrel. Specifically, patients taking these drugs are at increased risk for serious hemorrhagic events if a fall does occur.

There are also data to suggest that adding certain drugs to a medication regimen can decrease the risk of falling or associated complications. For example, in patients who fall frequently, calcium and vitamin D supplementation maintains bone health and improves muscle strength and tone, thereby reducing falls and fractures.[15]

The most common recommendations made by pharmacists at VA CT as part of fall consults are summarized in Table 18.6.

Interim Analysis

An interim analysis of the pharmacy fall-risk consult frequency was requested by the interdisciplinary team in the fall of 2006. This was due to an aggregate root cause analysis requested by the VISN (Vet-

Fall Interventions and Environmental Factors Used to Prevent Patient Falls

The following interventions and environmental factors can aid in preventing falls and should be implemented for all patients:

1. Orient the patient to his surroundings upon admission and when needed if cognitively impaired.
2. Demonstrate how to call for nurse or ring for assistance.
3. Instruct patient to call for help before getting out of bed or off stretcher.
4. Place bed/stretcher in lowest position when care is completed.
5. Use patient shoes or nonslip socks when getting patient out of bed.
6. Move tubing/wires out of the way for easier ambulation.
7. Inspect floor for wet areas and dry these areas.
8. Display the Environmentally Safe Patient Room Poster in a prominent area.
9. Place urine holders on beds/stretchers.
10. Maintain a clutter free environment, including bedside table, keeping items the patient uses frequently within reach.
11. Lock all wheelchairs and beds prior to moving patient.
12. Move legs on wheelchairs out of the way during transfer.
13. Assign patient to bed that allows him/her to exit on strong side.
14. Use transfer/lifting equipment/grab bars when moving patients.
15. Engage and instruct patient/significant other in all aspects of fall prevention.
16. Maintain proper lighting.
17. Inspect tips canes/walkers/crutches.
18. Instruct patients on how to use assistive devices prior to initiating them.
19. Instruct patients about side effects of medications and interactions with food or other supplements that may create fall risk.
20. Maintain awareness of changing symptoms or patient complaints that could precede a fall.
21. Provide rounds during meals, obtaining vital signs, and administering medication.

Additional Fall Interventions for High Risk In-Patients (Risk score >51)
1. Move the patient bed location close to nurses' station
2. Bed/chair alarm
3. Perimeter mattress (T3W)
4. Green armband and fall sticker placed on doorway
5. Toileting schedule
6. Communicate with other services about patient status for procedures or tests

Additional Fall Interventions for Low Risk In-Patients (Risk score 25–50)
1. Toileting schedule

Figure 18.1. Attachment C to Healthcare System Policy 118–015.

Table 18.6. Common Interventions Recommended by Pharmacy via Fall Consult

Adding hold parameters to the following:
    Cardiac medications
    Antihypertensives
    Hypoglycemics
    Insulin
    Sedatives

Changing to a hypnotic agent less likely to be implicated in a fall

Discontinuing drugs with questionable benefit

Changing dosing of sedating drugs to bedtime

Monitor for oversedation with sedatives

Therapeutic monitoring of narrow therapeutic index drugs

Pharmacokinetic and pharmacodynamic considerations

Reevaluate need for narcotic medications at current dose

Advise patient to stand slowly to avoid postural hypotension

Adding calcium and vitamin D supplementation to patients who fall

erans Integrated Service Network) in response to the NCPS and Joint Commission goals. The review of pharmacy fall-risk consult frequency determined that many of patients who were eligible for a pharmacy fall-risk consult did not actually have one requested by the nurse completing the intake/reassessment note. On closer review of the policy, the interdisciplinary team postulated that asking nurses to assess patient fall risk based on drug classes and symptoms may have been unreasonable. In reality, on the day of admission/transfer, nurses have multiple responsibilities; asking them to recognize the need for and initiate a pharmacy consult based on drug classes and symptoms was not reasonable.

To simplify the falls prevention measures at VA CT, the team changed the criteria for initiating a pharmacy fall-risk consult. The interdisciplinary team noticed that the criteria for entering a physical therapy consult were much simpler than entering a pharmacy consult. Rather than assessing the patient in more specific terms, a MFS score ≥50 alone would warrant a physical therapy consult. Specifically, hospital policy was revised so the criteria for a nurse to order a pharmacy consult would mirror the criteria for ordering a physical therapy consult: patients with an MFS score ≥50. This policy revision greatly simplified the process by which nurses determined whether a patient was eligible for this assessment.

The interim review compared the reporting of falls and pharmacy fall-risk consult requests prior to the initiation of the fall prevention program (Fiscal Year 2005) to the first two fiscal years the pharmacy fall consult service was in place (Fiscal Years 2006 and Fiscal Year 2007, quarters 1 through 3). Table 18.7 summarizes the findings.

After making the change in criteria for ordering a pharmacy fall-risk consult in the fall of 2006, there was a temporary increase in the frequency of pharmacy fall-risk consults during the fall and winter of 2006. Unfortunately, this increase in the pharmacy fall-risk consult was short lived. The team postulated there was some reduction in attention to detail regarding the fall policy as time passed. There also appeared to be some bias from the nursing staff against ordering pharmacy consults.

Table 18.7. Frequency of Falls before and after Initiation of Fall Prevention Program

	Fiscal Year 2005	Fiscal Year 2006	Fiscal Year 2007 Quarters 1–3
Consults completed	26	272	117
Falls reported	196	202	251

Multidisciplinary Team Recommendations

The interdisciplinary falls-risk team at VA CT is still actively pursuing interventions with patients, nurses, and physicians to increase awareness about the role of the pharmacist in reducing the risk of falls. The team continues to meet on a quarterly basis to review aggregate fall data and other pertinent fall-related issues. One recent recommendation included re-educating the staff regarding the necessity of requesting a pharmacy fall-risk consult for any patient who falls while admitted into the hospital, regardless of the MFS score. The interdisciplinary team is currently forming a work group to improve the current falls policy.

Other interventions recommended by the team include interdisciplinary fall prevention rounds, which occur weekly on each patient care unit. The goals of the fall prevention rounds are to observe the frequency and appropriateness of fall prevention measures, and for pharmacy staff to make recommendations to nurses and other members of the interdisciplinary care team to reduce patient risk for falling or harm resulting from falling. These rounds are supervised by the charge nurses on each ward. The general recommendations include ensuring environmental precautions are in place while identifying and removing safety hazards, and assigning staff to assist patients at high risk for falling. If any patterns are recognized via these weekly rounds, items for further intervention or followup are reported to the nurse manager of the ward and to the interdisciplinary fall team.[9]

Additionally, the nursing staff is responsible for placing green arm bands on all patients deemed high risk for falls, and orange stickers graphically representing fall risk are placed next to the patient's name outside the room. Further, patients at high risk for falling have been provided with chair or bed alarms such that nurses are made aware if the patient attempts to ambulate alone. For patients at high risk for falling, the nursing staff may perform patient checks at more frequent intervals, or provide one-to-one care for the most extreme cases.

Future Direction

This project is rapidly expanding. Currently, VA CT's postgraduate, year two, geriatric pharmacy specialty resident is working on a residency project evaluating whether clinical pharmacy intervention reduces the risk of repeat falls in hospitalized patients >65 years of age.

Furthermore, VA CT is investigating ways to increase the frequency of consults in patients who either fall or are at high risk for falling. The hospital's information technology specialists are working to determine whether the computerized patient record system is capable of automatically entering a consult if a post-fall note is entered for the patient. Secondly, the interdisciplinary team would like to have a pharmacy fall-risk consult ordered for any patient with an MFS score ≥50 automatically, without any additional nursing effort. This recommendation came from observations made during the interim review period.

Conclusions

VA CT was very proactive in addressing the Joint Commission's patient safety goal 9 to reduce the risk of harm resulting from falls. Unfortunately, the fall prevention program at VA CT has some weaknesses. Although the hospital has a simple, electronic mechanism for reporting falls, falls are not always reported, and the actual ordering of consults is not always completed. Fall data at VA CT lacks external validity in that the patient population is essentially male veterans. As previously mentioned, there is also the potential for subjectivity from the nursing staff regarding the utility of the pharmacy fall-risk consult service.

The implementation of a falls prevention policy and the development of an interdisciplinary fall-risk reduction program have now been in place for over 2 years. Members of the team have reviewed the data dealing with falls to evaluate the efficacy of the program. The patients deemed at high risk for falls were identified using the validated criteria of the MFS score. The computerized patient record system allowed for easy review of medication use that could increase fall risk. Hopefully, the lessons learned at VA CT can help other facilities address the Joint Commission goal of reducing patient harm resulting from falls.

References

1. Feder G, Cryer C, Donovan S, et al. Guidelines for the prevention of falls in people over 65. *BMJ.* 2000;321:1007-1011.

2. Kochanek KD, Murphy SL, Anderson RN, et al. Deaths: final data for 2002. *Natl Vital Stat Rep.* 2004;53(5):1-115.

3. Grisso JA, Kelsey JL, Strom BL, et al. Risk factors for falls as a cause of hip fracture in women. The Northeast Hip Fracture Study Group. *N Engl J Med.* 1991;324:1326-1331.

4. Leibson CL, Toteson ANA, Gabriel SE, et al. Mortality, disability, and nursing home use for persons with and without hip fracture: a population-based study. *J Am Geriatr Soc.* 2002;50:1644-1650.

5. Tinetti ME. Preventing falls in elderly persons. *N Engl J Med.* 2003;348:42-49.

6. Tinetti ME, Speechley M, Ginter SF, et al. Risk factors for falls among elderly persons living in the community. *N Engl J Med.* 1988;319:1701-1707.

7. The Joint Commission. 2005 hospital national patient safety goals. Available at: http://www.jointcommission.org/PatientSafety/NationalPatientSafetyGoals/05_hap_npsgs.htm.Accessed September 4, 2007.

8. VA National Center for Patient Safety. National Center for Patient Safety—falls toolkit. Available at: http://vaww.ncps.med.va.gov/Tools/fallstoolkit/index.html. Accessed July 12, 2007.

9. Veazey, MF. *VA Connecticut Healthcare System nursing policy CP-3 "Fall prevention."* West Haven, CT: Department of Veterans Affairs; 2005.

10. Morse JM, Morse RM, Tylko SJ. Development of a scale to identify the fall-prone patient. *Can J Aging.* 1989;8:366-377.

11. Agostini JV, Tinetti ME. Drugs and falls: rethinking the approach to medication risk in older adults. *J Am Geriatr Soc.* 2002;50:1744-1745.

12. Beers MH. Explicit criteria for determining potentially inappropriate medication use by the elderly: an update. *Arch Intern Med.* 1997;157:1531-1536.

13. Fick DM, Cooper JW, Wade WE, et al. Updating the Beers Criteria for potentially inappropriate medication use in older adults—results of a US consensus panel of experts. *Arch Intern Med.* 2003;163:2716-2724.

14. Walker PC, Alrawi A, Mitchell JF, et al. Medication use as a risk factor for falls among hospitalized elderly patients. *Am J Health Syst Pharm.* 2005;62:2495-2499.

15. Janssen HC, Samson MM, Verhaar HJ. Vitamin D deficiency, muscle function, and falls in elderly people. *Am J Clin Nutr.* 2002;75:611-615.

19

To Stock or Not to Stock Concentrated Epinephrine Multidose Vials in the Emergency Department (ED)

Joanne G. Kowiatek

Institution Description

The UPMC Presbyterian Hospital is a 647-bed, academic, not-for-profit medical center. It is part of the UPMC Health System (referred to as UPMC), which is located in western Pennsylvania. The UPMC Health System comprises 19 hospitals with 43,000 employees. UPMC also has a partnership with Palermo, Sicily to provide transplantation and other specialized international services.

UPMC Presbyterian is an adult medical/surgical referral hospital and a site of ongoing research and graduate programs in conjunction with the University of Pittsburgh School of Medicine and affiliated with the University of Pittsburgh, Schools of Health Sciences. The hospital offers organ transplantation, cardiology and cardiothoracic surgery, critical care medicine and trauma, psychiatry, rehabilitation, geriatrics, and neurosurgery services. UPMC Presbyterian is designated as a Level I Regional Resource Trauma Center.

Background

This chapter will review UPMC Presbyterian's process for ensuring safety when a hospital department, such as the emergency department (ED), requests medication(s) be added to floor stock. In 2003 based on medication safety alerts from the Institute for Safe Medication Practices (ISMP),[1,2] concentrated epinephrine multidose vials were removed from all automated medstations (automated medication storage and distribution devices) or floor stock and only stocked in emergency medication carts. These carts are used by the specialized and highly trained hospital medical emergency team (MET) members that respond to all recognized hospital emergencies.

Topical epinephrine for anterior nasal nosebleed (epistaxis), previously stocked in the ED, was commercially unavailable in 2005 due to a manufacturer shortage. The ED clinical staff requested an alternative, and, to management's surprise, a staff pharmacist actually recommended that the concentrated epinephrine 1 mg/mL (1:1000) injection 30-mL multidose vials be added to the ED automated medstation floor stock as an alternative to the commercially unavailable topical dosage form. Against pharmacy safety policy developed in 2003 based on the ISMP alerts,[1,2] and without pharmacy management approval, a staff pharmacist provided concentrated epinephrine injection as floor stock in the ED for topical use. This event occurred during the December 2005 holidays. This violation was discovered by the UPMC Presbyterian pharmacy manager of medication safety[3] (who reviews all requests that may relate to medication safety issues) when one of the pharmacy operations managers sent an e-mail asking the medication safety manager whether the concentrated injectable epinephrine was a safe alternative to the topical epinephrine and whether it was acceptable for the ED to stock. If not for this e-mail request, the safety intervention may have never occurred until a serious adverse event or medication error was reported.

Why Was an Intervention Necessary?

Intervention was necessary to ensure compliance with the existing pharmacy safety policy, which was developed based on national safety recommendations by the Joint Commission™ and the ISMP. The Joint Commission Medication Management Standard, MM.4.40 states: "Medications are dispensed safely." Joint Commission further requires that "medications are dispensed in the most ready-to-administer forms available from the manufacturer or if feasible, in unit-doses that have been repackaged by the pharmacy or licensed repackager." [4] The pharmacy had already decided that stocking the concentrated epinephrine injection 1 mg/mL (1:1000) on the patient units did not meet this Joint Commission safety standard. The ISMP notes national safety concerns with intravenous epinephrine as it is highly concentrated and has led to deaths and patient harm. [2,5-7] As part of the review for this safety initiative, a UPMC ear, nose, and throat (ENT) expert physician noted that there was the potential to give the concentrated epinephrine product accidentally by the intravenous route instead of the topical route, which is dangerous and prone to a fatal overdose. Then ENT expert physician noted no reason to use epinephrine topically in the treatment of epistaxis. He thought oxymetazoline solution worked very well and had a favorable safety profile. The ENT physician used it topically in the operating room and the outpatient ENT clinic. He was not a fan of topical lidocaine due to its slow onset of action. The ENT physician used topical pontocaine in the office though it has a narrower therapeutic range and noted that lidocaine or oxymetazoline could be applied separately or mixed together for epistaxis treatment in the ENT clinic. [8]

Recommended precautions for use of oxymetazoline, as provided by the pharmacy drug information center, were to avoid in patients receiving MAO inhibitors and to exercise caution in patients with coronary artery disease, hypertension, hyperthyroidism, and diabetes mellitus. (Note: This list of precautions may not be all inclusive.)

Epinephrine is considered a high-risk/high-alert medication as defined by the ISMP[9] and Joint Commission. The goal of this intervention was to enforce, reaffirm, and re-educate all staff regarding the existing policy: limit where concentrated epinephrine multidose vials were stocked to include only the pharmacy and emergency medication carts.

Intervention Description

The current "standard" safety review and decision process for floor stock medication requests may take several months, since it requires input from a variety of UPMC medication safety committees. However, the pharmacy management used the "expedited" version of this process to quickly respond to the request for the concentrated epinephrine multidose vials for injection to be added to the ED's floor stock. Specifically, the pharmacy management's assessment was that the request for concentrated epinephrine multidose vials to be added to the ED's floor stock required immediate action and resolution to ensure patient safety and that the appropriate medication for epistaxis patients was readily available. The expedited process included a review by an expert panel to determine the safety and risk versus patient benefit due to the unavailability of topical epinephrine for treatment of epistaxis. The panel involved the pharmacists from the drug information center who consulted with ENT physician experts for recommendations on safe and appropriate drug alternatives. The review also included a verification of compliance with Joint Commission Medication Management (MM) standards and with other national safety recommendations (e.g., ISMP recommendations). The process concluded with approval by an interdisciplinary group of UPMC Presbyterian physicians, pharmacists, and other hospital safety and quality personnel using an electronic mail discussion, and later by the formal approval process of the UPMC Presbyterian Safe Medication Practices and Quality Improvement (SMPQI) and Pharmacy and Therapeutics (P&T) committees. The goals of these discussions were education and involvement of physician staff and development of a plan to get information about the epinephrine safety initiative out to nursing staff as well as pharmacy and medical staffs.

The risk management and patient safety department was also very involved as representatives from this department sit on the UPMC Presbyterian SMPQI subcommittee. These individuals have an integral part in patient safety at UPMC, and participation in the SMPQI subcommittee keeps them informed of ongoing safety initiatives. UPMC Presbyterian's Department of Risk Management and Patient Safety supports physicians, nurses, pharmacists, and staff by working with them to prevent adverse outcomes related to pharmacotherapy and by analyzing those adverse events that do occur to implement improvements in patient care. This department reviews what occurs in these cases and uses that information to plan quality improvement initiatives for enhancing UPMC care, in collaboration with the pharmacy department.

Actions Taken

The following actions were taken, starting January 2006:

- UPMC Presbyterian approved oxymetazoline nasal spray (which was concluded to be safer than epinephrine) as the alternative drug of choice for epistaxis.
- The P&T committee decided topical epinephrine and concentrated intravenous epinephrine multidose vials were not to be stocked in the ED or in any patient unit or hospital department including the ENT outpatient clinic. The ENT outpatient clinic was not subject to the original policy, since the clinic is not hospital-based and, therefore, does not fall directly under the hospital's authority. However, UPMC Presbyterian's Department of Risk Management and Patient Safety helped enforce this particular decision at the clinic, since the ENT clinic is staffed by University of Pittsburgh physicians. These physicians fall under the scope of corporate risk management for the UPMC Health System.
- The pharmacy department sequestered all epinephrine concentrated 1 mg/mL (1:1000) injection 30-mL multidose vials inside an automated medstation in the pharmacy to track use/removal by all pharmacy staff, so that any removal and dispensing could be identified by staff members and questioned by pharmacy managers.
- Daily audit reports were run on the pharmacy automated medstation to check removal of epinephrine by pharmacy staff to ensure its use is only for emergency cart refill or for internal pharmacy use (e.g., admixing epinephrine infusions for patient unit).

Staff Education

This decision and its basis were communicated to all relevant clinicians, especially the ED clinical staff, outpatient ENT clinic staff, pharmacy staff, and other clinicians on inpatient units where epistaxis is a clinical concern. This decision was also reported to the ISMP to be shared nationally as appropriate. Once the topical epinephrine became commercially available again around February

2006, the P&T committee decided not to stock it in the hospital for any use and continued to use the oxymetazoline nasal spray for treatment of epistaxis cases.

Staff education occurred via various methods such as electronic mail and the train-the-trainers method (medical director to physician and resident staff, nurse director to nursing staff, and pharmacy director to pharmacy staff, and so on). Educational presentations were also made to various hospital safety committees, including the P&T committee and to the risk management and patient safety staff. The pharmacy director of the drug use and disease state management program[10] was key to physician education due to her positive relationship with the UPMC medical director who is a pharmacy champion. Information was shared with all 19 UPMC hospitals through presentations to the UPMC Health System P&T committee and the UPMC Health System Patient Safety committee. See Appendix 19.1 for an example of the educational tool that was sent to all clinical staff. The ISMP alerts related to epinephrine safety, mentioned in this chapter, were used for education as well.

Joint Commission Standards Impact

The impact of the safety initiative helps to ensure compliance with Joint Commission Medication Management standards, specifically related to Standard MM.4.40, which states: "Medications are dispensed safely."[4]

Outcome of Intervention

The goal of this intervention was to limit where the concentrated epinephrine multidose vials were stocked to only the pharmacy department and the emergency medication carts. There were only two known (reported) policy violations, since this new process was implemented in January 2006, where concentrated epinephrine was left outside of an opened emergency cart, unsecured by nursing staff and "stashed" in their medication room. These incidents were discovered by alert pharmacists and pharmacy technician staff (medication safety technicians) who were educated on this safety issue. Once reported to the pharmacy manager of medication safety and to the risk management department as a medication event and potential medication error, the unit director of the patient unit was alerted and the nursing staff on that unit was re-educated as to hospital policies and safety issues regarding concentrated epinephrine vials.

No actual medication errors have occurred involving this high-alert medication before or after this intervention was implemented and as of August 2007. The pharmacy management and pharmacy medication safety team members continue to track removal of concentrated epinephrine vials from the pharmacy automated medstation to ensure safe and appropriate use and to track where the vials are being used (e.g., vials may be removed for use in the pharmacy sterile products area for admixing intravenous infusions). Pharmacy staff members are questioned, if unsure, where vials are dispensed, why vials are needed, and who outside the pharmacy requests them. This questioning provides opportunities for external and internal staff re-education.

Lessons Learned

One lesson learned via negative feedback was that the pharmacy decision team forgot to include a key physician in the outpatient ENT clinic. This physician requested the concentrated epinephrine multidose vials several months after all of the decisions to remove them from general availability were made. Due to this medication stock request, the ENT physician learned of the recent decision and was very upset that he/she was not included in the initial discussion due to his/her expertise with epistaxis. Unfortunately, this physician and his/her expertise were overlooked as he/she had a greater presence in the outpatient clinic setting and not in the inpatient setting so was not as well-known to pharmacy leadership. The pharmacy manager of medication safety apologized and explained the decision and its basis (including national safety recommendations that guided this change), and the physician agreed with it, although he/she was offended at not being initially included in the decision-making process.

A second lesson learned was that the nursing staff at UPMC Presbyterian adjusted their practice, creating a workaround to meet their needs, not always understanding the safety problems they created. For example, nurses in the intensive care units (ICU) would remove the concentrated epinephrine multidose vials from the emergency medication carts after the cart was opened for an emergency and before the cart was sent to the pharmacy for exchange and medication replacement. The nurses' reasoning was that they wanted to have the epinephrine vials available for admixing intravenous infusions when they were needed, obviating the need to call pharmacy for admixing the infusion and reducing the delay. This unsafe practice was detected by a pharmacy medication safety technician during a routine monthly pharmacy inspection.

Recommended Actions for Lessons Learned

- Lesson 1: Prevent the omission of key physicians from medication safety decisions by checking with as many different disciplines and clinicians as possible. Include both inpatient and outpatient hospital-based patient care areas and the hospital administration as well. It still may be possible to overlook key individuals. If such an oversight occurs, education and apologies should be made to keep a positive and cooperative working environment focused on patient safety.

- Lesson 2: Though not always easy, anticipate both pharmacy and nursing staff workarounds that may bypass patient safety for the sake of convenience. It is important to anticipate possible breaches in practice and determine why shortcuts are being taken. Once the root issue is determined then preventative measures may be put into place. In this case nursing staff did not believe the pharmacy could provide the epinephrine infusions in a timely manner so the pharmacy operations management had to resolve this turnaround time concern with the ICU nursing staffs and directors. Currently, with the help of the unit-based pharmacists and pharmacy technicians, as well as the monthly pharmacy inspections performed by the pharmacy medication safety technicians, epinephrine hoarding has declined and is better monitored.

Updates and Changes

During routine pharmacy monitoring of the concentrated epinephrine vials stored in the pharmacy automated medstation, several deviations from the newly established procedures were found and the tracking process allowed the pharmacy managers to determine which pharmacist removed the vials and where they were sent. For example, in June 2006 a pharmacist removed a vial to be sent to the postanesthesia care unit automated medstation. When questioned, the pharmacist was not aware of the safety initiative in place and was educated. At this time a reminder e-mail was sent to all pharmacy staff. In general with safety initiatives, it is good to send periodic reminders to catch any new staff hired since the initiative was put into place. To date no other changes have been put into place for this safety initiative.

Summary

To ensure patient safety, educate all pharmacy staff to bring all new or unusual medication floor stock requests to pharmacy management and the medication safety manager (or other pharmacy personnel as appropriate) for their review and approval. There can never be enough education related to medication safety initiatives so continued vigilance is essential. Also, use of pharmacy technician staff and medication safety technicians to detect unsafe practices is an asset to medication safety.

References

1. Institute for Safe Medication Practices. *ISMP Medication Safety Alert.* April 17, 2003. "Looks" like a problem: ephedrine—epinephrine. Available at: http://www.ismp.org/newsletters/acutecare/articles/20030417_2.asp. Accessed August 14, 2007.

2. Institute for Safe Medication Practices. *ISMP Medication Safety Alert.* December 4, 1996. Case update: epinephrine death in Florida. Available at: Available at: http://www.ismp.org/newsletters/acutecare/ articles/19961204.asp. Accessed August 14, 2007.

3. Kowiatek JG, Weber RJ, Skeldar SJ, et al. Medication safety manager in an academic medical center. *Am J Health Syst Pharm.* 2004;61:58-64.

4. The Joint Commission: *2007 Comprehensive Accreditation Manual for Hospitals: The Official Handbook.* Oakbrook Terrace, IL: Joint Commission Resources, 2006.

5. Institute for Safe Medication Practices. *ISMP Medication Safety Alert.* August 12, 2004. ISMP petitions USP on epinephrine issues. Available at: http://www.ismp.org/Newsletters/acutecare/ articles/20040812.asp?ptr=y. Accessed August 14, 2007.

6. Institute for Safe Medication Practices. *ISMP Medication Safety Alert.* October 16, 2002. It doesn't pay to play the percentages. Available at: http://www.ismp.org/Newsletters/acutecare/ articles/20021016.asp?ptr=y. Accessed August 14, 2007.

7. Institute for Safe Medication Practices. ISMP advocates changes in epinephrine labeling. Available at: http://www.ismp.org/pressroom/PR20040812.pdf. Accessed August 14, 2007.

8. Nasal Emergencies and Sinusitis. Table 241-1. Vasoconstrictive and anesthetic agents used in epistaxis. In: Tintinalli JE, Kelen GD, Stapczynski JS, eds. *Emergency Medicine: A Comprehensive Study Guide,* 6th Edition. New York: The McGraw-Hill Companies; 2004:Chapter 241.

9. Cohen MR, Kilo M. High-alert medications: safeguarding against errors. In Cohen MR, ed. *Medication Errors.* Washington, DC: American Pharmaceutical Association; 1999:5.1-5.40.

10. Skledar SJ, Hess MM. Implementation of a drug-use and disease-state management program. *Am J Health Syst Pharm.* 2000;57(suppl.):23S-29S.

Appendix 19.1. UPMC Epinephrine Medication Safety Alert

Medication Safety Alert! DO NOT dispense epinephrine 1 mg/mL 30 mL multidose vial (MDV) to any unit or staff member.

Safe Treatment of Nose Bleeds

Due to the current unavailability of a previously commercially marketed <u>topical</u> epinephrine product, there have been requests for pharmacy to dispense the **concentrated IV epinephrine 1:1000 (1 mg/mL) 30 mL MDV dose vial** to the ED and other inpatient units for epistaxis (nosebleeds). Use of the **IV epinephrine** for this purpose poses a **serious safety concern,** based on national and local medication events (**see links at bottom of e-mail**). **Use of IV epinephrine topically in the treatment of epistaxis is potentially dangerous and prone to overdosing.** Though the request has been for topical use, IV Epinephrine could easily be inadvertently injected IV and cause **serious harm or death.**

After discussion with an ENT specialist, it was determined that **oxymetazoline** (Afrin, Genasal) solution is the appropriate agent for treatment of epistaxis (nose bleeds). **Oxymetazoline is a topical decongestant that acts as a local vasoconstrictor, and may be useful when applied prior to pinching the nose. It may be effectively applied by soaking cotton balls with the solution and inserting them into the nose on the side of hemorrhage.**

Possible adverse events associated with oxymetazoline include palpitations, lightheadedness, and burning of mucous membranes.

Use of oxymetazoline (Afrin®, Genasal®, etc.) should be avoided in patients receiving Monoamine Oxidase (MAO) inhibitors, and caution should be exercised in patients with coronary artery disease, hypertension, hyperthyroidism, and diabetes mellitus.

Because of the availability of this safe and effective alternative to epinephrine, the **pharmacy should NOT dispense concentrated epinephrine to inpatient units when the intended use is for topical administration in a patient with a nose bleed. Oxymetazoline should be recommended as an alternative.**

EPINEPHRINE safety concerns are noted in the following articles:

http://www.ismp.org/Newsletters/acutecare/articles/20040812.asp?ptr=y;

http://www.ismp.org/Newsletters/acutecare/articles/19961204.asp?pt

http://www.ismp.org/Newsletters/acutecare/articles/20021016.asp?ptr=y;

http://www.ismp.org/pressroom/PR20040812.pdf

This alert is being sent on behalf of the Drug Information Center, Drug Use and Disease State Management, and Pharmacy Manager of Medication Safety. (Note: The information in this alert may not be all inclusive.)

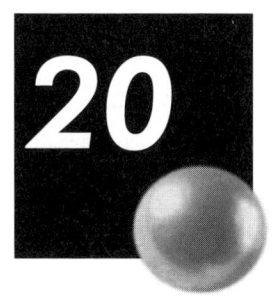

20

The Magical Medication Flowchart: Surmounting Barriers to Quality of Care in the Ambulatory Care Clinic

Angela R. Vinti

Acknowledgments:

Joanne Connaughton-Storey, MD; Regina Halecky, RN; Karen Acello, RN; and Patricia Cardano, Mercy Fitzgerald Outpatient Medical Clinic/Ambulatory Care, Darby, Pennsylvania

Huyla G. Coker, Pharm.D., The University of North Carolina at Chapel Hill School of Pharmacy, Elizabeth City State Satellite Campus, Elizabeth City, North Carolina

Martha W. Jones, Pharm.D., Scotland Neck Family Medical Center, Scotland Neck, North Carolina

Introduction

Medication reconciliation is defined by the Institute for Healthcare Improvement (IHI) as "creating the most accurate list possible of all medications a patient is taking—including drug name, dosage, frequency, and route—and comparing that list against the physician's admission, transfer, and/or discharge orders with the goal of providing correct medications to the patient at all transition points within the hospital."[1] You may ask, "How does this definition accurately reflect the need for medication reconciliation in an ambulatory care clinic?" Hospital-based ambulatory care clinics are part of the hospital system, and, as such, are required to work toward accreditation standards and goals set by The Joint Commission™ in order for the entire hospital system to be successful in the accreditation process. Medication reconciliation has been established as Goal 8 in the Joint Commission Ambulatory Care and Office-Based Surgery National Patient Safety Goals (NPSG), first announced in July 2004. The goal for 2008 reads:

> "Goal 8: Accurately and completely reconcile medications across the continuum of care. 8A: There is a process for comparing the patient's current medications with those ordered for the patient while under the care of the organization. 8B: A complete list of the patient's medications is communicated to the next provider of service when a patient is referred or transferred to another setting, service, practitioner or level of care within or outside the organization. The complete list of medications is also provided to the patient on discharge from the facility."[2]

While it may still seem that a hospital-based ambulatory care clinic is not subject to these standards, there may be circumstances within the clinic, which would legitimize its place within NPSG 8 and trigger the need for the clinic to develop a medication reconciliation process. For example, the hospital-based ambulatory care clinic may be located in a small, community-based teaching hospital, which has many interns, residents, and attending physicians rotating through the clinic. This scenario would constitute a "transition" or "transfer" of care within this setting, primarily because a patient may not see the same provider at every point of service.

Solutions for medication reconciliation have been implemented for inpatient facilities. Many of these solutions are electronic and require financial commitment, as well as technological support. Financial and technological resources may be difficult to come by for the small, community- and hospital-based ambulatory care clinics that lack electronic medical records. These challenges present quite a conundrum in keeping up to speed with medication reconciliation in the outpatient setting.

This chapter describes a process by which the medication reconciliation needs of a hospital-based ambulatory care clinic were identified and a tool was created and implemented to address those needs.

The Setting

Mercy Fitzgerald Hospital is a 368-bed, acute care, community teaching hospital serving Delaware County and Southwest Philadelphia. The ambulatory care services/clinic affiliated with the institution is located in the Sister Marie Lenahan Mercy Wellness Center, located on the Mercy Fitzgerald Hospital campus in Darby, Pennsylvania. The clinic census is approximately 3,000 patients per year.* Patient visits are scheduled Monday through Thursday, afternoons hours only; each weekday has an assigned attending physician, as well as five assigned resident and intern physicians. Patients are encouraged to schedule visits on the same weekday throughout their care to allow the intern, resident, and attending physicians to provide some continuity of care to the patient; however, this recommendation is not always followed by patients. In addition, intern and resident assignments to specialized inpatient care units dictate whether those personnel will be fulfilling clinic duties for a month(s) at a time, which opens the door for the transitioning of patients from one medical professional to another on a monthly basis. Documentation in the clinic is accomplished through a paper charting system where interns, residents, and attending physicians are required to document visits in their own handwriting at the point of care. The clinic is supported by one receptionist, one full-time nurse (who is also the head administrator for the clinic), one part-time nurse, and a newly introduced pharmacy practice faculty member from a local college of pharmacy. This pharmacist has expertise in ambulatory care/chronic disease state management and began supporting/integrating into the clinic in August 2005.

Identifying a Need (Objectives)

With the introduction of a pharmacy practice faculty member, it was important for this individual to assess the needs of the clinic regarding medication management and respond to those needs. Needs of the clinic were assessed through casual conversations with support staff, the medical director of the clinic, attending physicians, and resident and intern physicians. Conversations with support staff uncovered the fact that over 10 telephone calls per half-day of clinic were received from patients whose main concerns were to report and/or discuss medication-related issues. These issues included nonformulary medications being prescribed by the clinic physicians, side effect reporting, socioeconomic considerations, confusion over discontinued medications, questions on how to use

---

*The census figure was obtained from the clinic administrator, who tracks patient visits through the billing department.

devices that were prescribed, and requests for refills or new medications. The nurse administrator was also concerned with meeting Joint Commission standards in regards to patient safety. Being a hospital-based clinic, the documentation of patient care in the clinic is continuously open to Joint Commission review for adherence to standards. The nurse administrator was concerned that medication documentation was not adequate for the NPSG 8 in regards to medication reconciliation. Discussions with intern and resident physicians revealed frustration in seeing new patients every week who might subsequently be transitioned from one intern/resident to another; confusion surrounding antiquated documentation of patients' medications and allergies in the paper medical chart; reluctance to authorize refills due to lack of familiarity with patients' medication regimens; and the limited time that was available for discussing medication changes and proper usages during patient visits. The clinic's medical director and other attending physicians in the practice echoed the intern and resident physicians' concerns and expressed some of their own. The attending physicians were concerned with the sources of medication documentation. To them, it seemed as if patients were unreliable due to cognitive impairment or purposeful deception. Many attending physicians specifically cited two scenarios: 1) patients were being referred from the hospital's emergency room with a diagnosis of nonmalignant pain and were supposedly being told that the clinic physicians would indiscriminately write prescriptions for opioid analgesics, and 2) patients histories, regardless of medications prescribed, reflected multiple pharmacies providing their medications. Throughout the dialog with vested parties, there was also concern on the part of the medical director and nurse administrator that the attending resident and intern physicians may not understand the role or the intent of the pharmacy practice faculty member in the clinic.

In her own assessment of patient charts, the pharmacy practice faculty member noticed that there was not a consistent method of medication documentation. All charts had medications documented in a small section, approximately 1" high and 7" wide, on a face-sheet. These face-sheets listed disease states and regular health maintenance information as well (e.g., immunization status and dates administered). A detailed look at the medications listed on the face-sheets revealed that the dates associated with them were consistently at least 2 years old and contained dangerous abbreviations as identified by the Institute for Safe Medication Practices (ISMP), such as "Zestril 10 mg PO qd, 2/10/2003." Within the providers' notes for each chart, intern and resident physicians documented patients' medications inconsistently—some physicians documented at each visit, while others did not document medications at all. The patient notes that did contain medication documentation were incomplete—only listing either brand or generic name, and lacking documentation of drug dose, route, frequency, and any compliance information. Patient notes that did not contain medication documentation either did not contain any information on medications at all or referred to the face-sheet for information on patients' current medications.

After a month of conversations, observations, and reflections on the concerns of all parties involved in the operations of the clinic, the medical director, nurse administrator, and the pharmacy practice faculty member determined that following needs/goals existed and were to be addressed:

1. Reducing medication-related phone calls to reception/administration
2. Reducing dispensing, dosing, drug choice, and transcription errors
3. Educating patients on their medications
4. Documenting medications, regimen changes, and medication allergies over time
5. Providing consistent documentation to varying resident staff
6. Educating providers on the role of the pharmacy practice faculty member
7. Integrating the pharmacy practice faculty member into the daily operations of the clinic

Ultimately, addressing all these needs would improve the quality and continuity of care for the patients in the clinic. Need/goal number 4 seemed to be the root of all others. It was apparent that the task to be undertaken was developing and implementing a mode of efficient, comprehensive, and accurate medication documentation that is able to span across a continuum of time. The clinic needed to develop and implement its own method of continuous and repetitive medication reconciliation. Who would be accountable for this? Why, the pharmacy practice faculty member, of course!

Creating and Implementing a Solution (Methods)

With the adoption of the clinic's lofty goal, the pharmacy practice faculty member turned to her residency training experience where she functioned in similar environment—a small, community hospital-based clinic with a paper charting system and trainees rotating through the practice site. In these types of settings, a form of documentation known as the *medication flowchart* was used to document patients' medications, allergies, and changes to medication regimens over time. From memory, the pharmacy practice faculty member re-created this documentation in electronic format and presented the potential solution to the medical director and nurse administrator. Suggestions were made to include more fields for properly identifying the patient (e.g., a field was added for Date of Birth in addition to Medical Record Number, and a final product was then produced, see Figure 20.1). Questions still remained: "Where would this document get placed in the chart?" "How would it be easily recognized by all?" "Who would be accountable for completing the documentation?" "How often should the documentation be completed?" "How long should the process take?" "How can the most accurate information be gathered on the flowchart?" "Should this flowchart be put in all charts or just selected patients?"

In addition to NPSG 8, Joint Commission provides recommendations that healthcare organizations consider "placing the medication list in a highly visible location in the patient's chart, and including dosage, drug schedules, immunizations, and allergies or drug intolerances on the list."[2] Joint Commission also recommends "creating a process for reconciling medications at all interfaces of care and determining reasonable time frames for reconciling medications. Patients, responsible physicians, nurses, and pharmacists should be involved in the medication reconciliation process."[2] Taking these recommendations into consideration, the clinic staff began to answer many of its own questions. It was decided that the medication flowchart was to be produced on pastel green paper and placed at the front of each patient chart, on the left-hand side of the chart, directly underneath the one-page patient face-sheet that lists disease states and regular health maintenance information.

To begin, the implementation of the medication flowchart initiative was championed by the pharmacy practice faculty member. This allowed the individual to have an easily identifiable role in the clinic for providers to identify with and call upon. In addition, this flowchart and medication reconciliation process provided Pharm.D. students on rotation with the faculty member the opportunity to interact with patients on a daily basis. Since the pharmacy practice faculty member and the Pharm.D. students would begin the implementation of this process, it was decided that not every patient on every single clinic day could be interviewed for the purpose of completing the medication flowchart. Therefore, daily patient schedules were prescreened to identify those patients who had diagnoses of chronic disease states. These were the patients who were given priority on any given clinic day to have an interview with the pharmacy practice faculty member or the Pharm.D. students. Patients who were not flagged for chronic disease states were also given the opportunity to go through the medication reconciliation process, at the availability of an interviewer(s). The ultimate goal for the entire census of patients at the ambulatory care clinic was 100% medication reconciliation documentation on the medication flowchart.

The pharmacy practice faculty member and Pharm.D. students would begin the medication

Mercy Fitzgerald Ambulatory Care Clinic—Medication Flowchart MR#: _____

Patient Name: _____   DOB: _____   Phone: _____

Pharmacy Name: _____   Phone: _____

Allergies: _____

MEDICATION	Date⇨ Initials⇨								

Figure 20.1. Blank Medication Flowchart Used at the Mercy Fitzgerald Ambulatory Care Clinic. The original document fits 8.5"x11" paper, uses 10-point Arial font, with 1" top, 0.5" bottom, and 0.75" side margins.

reconciliation process by entering patient exam rooms, introducing themselves, identifying their purpose, and requesting permission to proceed with the process. No patient refused this opportunity. Questions asked during the medication reconciliation process included, but were not limited to, "What is the name of the medication you take?" "What strength is the medication?" "How do you take the medication?" "How often do you take the medication?" "What special directions do you follow when taking this medication?" "What is the medication for?" All of these questions not only allowed for gathering of information by the interviewer, but also opened windows of opportunity to provide patient education on any number of important issues.

The most reliable information was obtained during interviews when patients brought their medication bottles to the clinic with them; however, these circumstances were few and far between. To increase this occurrence and the reliability of the medication reconciliation process, signs were posted at key places in the clinic waiting area, patient rooms, triage station, and restrooms, reminding patients to "PLEASE BRING ALL MEDICATION BOTTLES TO EACH VISIT." Regardless of the presence of prescription bottles, after all patient interviews, permission was requested to telephone all patients' community pharmacies in order to verify information reported by the patient and/or caregiver. Not one patient or caregiver protested this procedure.

The initial process of completing the medication flowchart was the most time-consuming portion of the longitudinal medication reconciliation process. Initial patient interviews took up to 20 minutes at times, which frustrated some of the providers who were eager to conduct their own patient interviews and present to the attending physician. Once the initial medication flowchart was completed, updates to the document were required at every subsequent patient visit. Depending on the number of medications a patient was taking and the number of specialist providers a patient might see, interviews for the medication flowchart updates took anywhere from 5 to 15 minutes. In addition, interview times had the propensity to increase if patients were comfortable enough with the interviewer to ask questions about medication-related issues and/or report side effects. Once complete assessments of patients' medications and allergies were documented on the medication flowchart, this information was presented to the intern or resident physicians prior to their interviewing patients. At the conclusion of patient visits in the clinic, the pharmacy practice faculty member and Pharm.D. students would consult with the interns and residents to ensure that all medication changes were accurately documented on the medication flowchart.

A typical medication flowchart may look like Figure 20.2. For each patient visit, the individual conducting the medication reconciliation process and filling out the medication flowchart puts the date and his/her initials at the top of a column. During subsequent medication flowchart updates, this indicates to all other parties on what date the previous medication reconciliation process was completed and who completed the process, respectively. The individual conducting the initial patient interview lists all patient medications in the column on the far left of the flowchart. As medications get added to a patient's regimen, subsequent personnel will add the names of medications to the far left column. Individuals conducting the medication reconciliation interview and updating the medication flowchart use a variety of symbols to indicate continuations and changes in drug therapy over time. $\rightarrow$ signifies continuation of a medication, its dose, route, and frequency. $\uparrow$ signifies an increase in medication dose or frequency. $\downarrow$ signifies a decrease in medication dose or frequency. Rx + _R signifies that a prescription was either written or called in to the pharmacy at that particular visit with the corresponding number of refills authorized. D/C signifies the discontinuation of a medication. A box with an X through it signifies that the medication was not prescribed to the patient at that particular point in time. The word *Start* signifies the initiation of therapy with a particular medication at that point in time. Upon a new visit/update to the medication flowchart, providers and participants in the medication reconciliation process must refer to all dose and/or frequency changes to accurately assess what medication dose and frequency a patient should currently be taking.

Over time, the information on the medication flowcharts proved useful to the physicians in resolving patient problems, including, but not limited to, uncontrolled disease states, disease states not documented, and medication samples from a specialty provider's office. Physicians began to seek out medication flowchart information from the pharmacy practice faculty member and Pharm.D. students, in addition to wanting to participate in the process themselves. When physicians began asking

Mercy Fitzgerald Ambulatory Care Clinic—Medication Flowchart MR#: 001122

Patient Name: Michael Smith DOB: 01/01/1960 Phone: 610-555-0123

Pharmacy Name: Walgreens (Springfield) Phone: 610-555-4567

Allergies: Penicillin (hives), aspirin (anaphylaxis)

Date ⇨ MEDICATION Initials ⇨	2/9/07 ARV	4/29/07 KA	6/7/07 ARV	9/15/07 FK	
Lisinopril 20 mg PO qdaily	→	↑ to 40 mg Rx +2R	→	→	
Avapro 300 mg PO qdaily	→	→	→	→	
HCTZ 12.5 mg PO qdaily	→	→	→	→	
Metformin 500 mg 2 tabs PO BID	Rx + 2R	→	↓ to 1 tab	→	
Paroxetine 20 mg PO qdaily	→	→	D/C		
Loratadine 10 mg PO qdaily prn allergies		Start Rx + 3R	→	→	
Cymbalta 30 mg PO at bedtime			Start Rx + 0R	↑ to 60 mg Rx + 2R	
Humulin 70/30 Inject 12 units SUBQ BID				Start Rx + 0R	
Plavix 75 mg PO qdaily				Start Rx + 5R	

Figure 20.2. Example Medication Flowchart Used at the Mercy Fitzgerald Ambulatory Care Clinic. For illustrative purposes, the number of columns and rows in this figure are less than the actual medication flowchart used in the clinic setting (see Figure 20.1).

how and if they could participate in using the medication reconciliation form, that was the impetus for providing education to the physicians on the rationale and procedure for using the medication flowchart to reconcile patients' medications longitudinally. One-on-one education and training was provided by the pharmacy practice faculty member to the interested provider. The education and training of all providers was completed over a period of 2–3 months. Repetition of the training and assistance in filling out the flowchart was required while physician staff became accustomed to the medication reconciliation process. Gradually, the intern and resident physicians took the lead.

Were the Needs Met? (Results and Discussion)

Were the needs of the clinic met? There is a multifaceted answer to this question. Most of the aforementioned needs will be examined individually, with the remainder being examined collectively.

1. *Reducing medication-related phone calls to reception/administration.* This goal was met. Immediately following the implementation of the medication reconciliation process, the clinic secretarial and nursing staff reported a decrease in the number telephone calls from patients regarding medication refill requests, side effect concerns, and other general medication questions. The staff also reported a decrease in the number of phone calls from pharmacies in regards to nonformulary drug choices, potential drug-drug interactions, and socioeconomic concerns of the patients.

2. *Reducing dispensing, dosing, drug choice, and transcription errors.* It is difficult to determine if this need was met. While it is known that the medication reconciliation process provided a forum for increasing accuracy of patients' medication regimens, there is no objective documentation collated to show that these errors were reduced. The pharmacy practice faculty member can report that physicians asked more questions of her in order to verify dosing, directions, and choice of therapeutic agent.

3. *Educating patients on their medications.* This goal was met and is evidenced in the decreased number of phone calls to the front end secretarial and nursing staff, as well as the inherent opportunities for discussing the purpose of each medication during the medication reconciliation process/interview.

4. *Documenting medications, regimen changes, and medication allergies over time.* This goal was met. Documentation began with and was consistent and reliable among the pharmacy practice faculty member and Pharm.D. students. Once the process expanded to include the intern and resident physicians, the process became less consistent and less reliable. Regardless of the ease of use of the medication flowchart, some intern and resident physicians did not document and update the flowcharts as consistently as others. There could be any number of reasons for the observed lack of documentation. These reasons would be expected to vary (and would need to be further investigated) at any individual clinic that chooses to implement this kind of process.

5. *Providing consistent documentation to varying resident staff.* Again, this need was met at first with the advent of the documentation being performed by pharmacy personnel, but without re-educating and retraining the medical personnel involved in the process, documentation became inconsistent, once again.

6. *Educating providers on the role of the pharmacy practice faculty member and integrating the pharmacy practice faculty member into the daily operations of the clinic.* It is entirely possible that these goals were met. Once the medication reconciliation process was in place and the medication flowchart was being utilized by the physician staff, questions began to arise for the pharmacy faculty member to address. Patient cases were discussed and drug choices were influenced by the clinical, practical, and economics information the pharmacy practice faculty member had to offer.

Many of the assessments of the needs/goals are entirely subjective and purely observational. With more foresight, the clinic could have collected more objective information for reporting purposes and potentially made more of an impact on the literature surrounding medication reconciliation in the outpatient setting. For example, the number of telephone calls per day to the ambulatory care clinic could have been recorded before, during, and after the full implementation of the medication reconciliation process.

The medication flowchart is for the documentation of chronic medications only, not acute or short-course medications, such as oral antibiotics for an acute sinus infection. Acute or short-course medications are not included on this form with the intention that those medications should be prescribed to a patient based on the chronic disease states and medications that he/she is already taking. It is essential to document these acute/short-course medications in patients' progress notes, but the documentation of these medications uses critical space on the medication flowchart, which should be reserved for longitudinal medication tracking. In addition, when acute or short-course medications are documented on the list along with other chronic medications, it conveys an unclear message to the provider that a patient may be taking a short-course medication on a chronic basis, particularly if the medication flowchart is not updated properly to reflect a discontinuation in that acute or short-course medication. Some may believe that not including acute or short-course medications in the medication flowchart documentation is a limitation, but it is certainly an opportunity for improvement of the documentation.

Conclusion

Many hospital-based, ambulatory care clinics in small, community-based teaching hospitals face challenges in the realm of medication reconciliation. These challenges may involve continuously transitioning personnel, lack of an electronic medical record, or lack of financial support for implementing a computerized process for medication reconciliation, just to name a few. It is essential for these clinics to develop medication reconciliation processes through which they can meet NPSG 8 and contribute to the successful accreditation of the institution. Such a process needs to have the buy-in of the clinic administrators and staff. Implementation can begin with the pharmacy personnel only or as a collaborative effort among all disciplines. Regardless of how the process begins, re-education of all parties involved in the process is essential to ensure that medication reconciliation is being done consistently for all patients. For the continued success of such an initiative, it would be essential to examine medication flowchart documentation for specific patterns or trends and report findings to the medical and other healthcare personnel involved on a routine basis. This retrospective evaluation would inherently be a quality assurance mechanism and provide a forum for addressing any barriers to the success of the medication reconciliation process and areas for improvement.

References

1. Institute for Healthcare Improvement. Campaign Overview. http://www.ihi.org/IHI/Programs/Campaign/Campaign.htm?TabId=1. Accessed July 30, 2007.
2. The Joint Commission. 2008 Ambulatory Care and Office-Based Surgery Programs National Patient Safety Goals. Available at: http://www.jointcommission.org/PatientSafety/NationalPatientSafetyGoals/08_amb_obs_npsgs.html. Accessed July 30, 2007.

Resources

Barnsteiner JH. Medication reconciliation: transfer of medication information across settings-keeping it free from error. *Am J Nurs.* March 2005;(suppl):31S-36S.

Bartick M, Baron D. Medication reconciliation at Cambridge Health Alliance. *Am J Med Qual.* 2006;21:304-306.

Boockvar KS, LaCorte HC, Giambanco V, et al. Medication reconciliation for reducing drug-discrepancy adverse events. *Am J Geriatr Pharmacother.* 2006;4:236-243.

Endo J, Jacobsen K. Medication reconciliation in Wisconsin: insights from a local initiative. *Wisconsin Medical Journal.* 2006;105:42-44.

Hayes BD, Donovan JL, Smith BS, et al. Pharmacist-conducted medication reconciliation in an emergency department. *Am J Health Syst Pharm.* 2007;64:1720-1723.

Ketchum K, Grass CA, Padwojski A. Medication reconciliation: verifying medication orders and clarifying discrepancies should be standard practice. *Am J Nurs.* 2005;105:78-85.

Levanda M. Implementing a medication reconciliation process in a community hospital. *Am J Health Syst Pharm.* 2007;64:1372-1378.

Manno MS, Hayes DD. How medication reconciliation saves lives. *Nursing.* 2006;36:63-64.

Poon EG, Blumenfeld B, Hamann C, et al. Design and implementation of an application and associated services to support interdisciplinary medication reconciliation efforts at an integrated healthcare delivery network. *J Am Med Inform Assoc.* 2006;13:581-592.

Sievers B, Wolf S. Achieving clinical nurse specialist competencies and outcomes through interdisciplinary education. *Clin Nurse Spec.* 2006;20:75-80.

Varkey P, Cunningham J, Bisping S. Improving medication reconciliation in the outpatient setting. *Jt Comm J Qual Patient Saf.* 2007;33:286-292.

Varkey P, Reller MK, Smith A, et al. An experimental interdisciplinary quality improvement education initiative. *Am J Med Qual.* 2006;21:317-322.

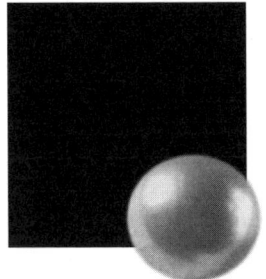

Index